IT'S A
SMALL WORLD
AFTER ALL

Life under The Microscope

JESPER LEONARD VUN

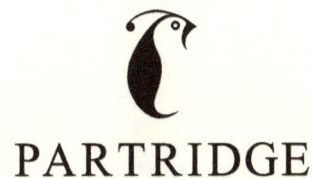

PARTRIDGE

ISBN:	Hardcover	978-1-5437-6499-4
	Softcover	978-1-5437-6497-0
	eBook	978-1-5437-6498-7

Reviewed by:

Jessica Sushma D'Souza
MSc Medical Microbiology (MAHE); PhD Scholar (MAHE)
Selection Grade Lecturer
Department of Microbiology, Manipal University College Malaysia (MUCM), Manipal, India

Print information available on the last page.

To order additional copies of this book, contact
Toll Free +65 3165 7531 (Singapore)
Toll Free +60 3 3099 4412 (Malaysia)
orders.singapore@partridgepublishing.com

www.partridgepublishing.com/singapore

Graphic artist: Jesper Leonard Vun Kien Fung

To my beloved parents,

Joseph & Freda

whose curiosity fuelled my motivation

CONTENTS

Foreword... xi

Preface..xiii

Introduction.. xvii

Chapter 1   The Basic Unit of Life 1

Chapter 2   The Body's Defences 10

Chapter 3   A Vaccine in Time Saves Nine........................22

Chapter 4   A Place for Everything, Everything in its Place 31

Chapter 5   An Introduction to Infection..........................37

Chapter 6   Basic Bacteriology...................................43

     Part 1: Characteristics of Bacteria 44
     Part 2: Classification of Bacteria 50
     Part 3: Bacterial Reproduction and Growth Curve 55
     Part 4: Medically Significant Bacteria...................58
     Part 5: How Antibiotics Work 67
     Basic Bacteriology Summary...........................71

Chapter 7   Basic Mycology 73

     Part 1: Characteristics of Fungi 74
     Part 2: Classification of Fungi..........................78

Part 3: Medically Significant Fungi 81
Part 4: How Antifungal Drugs Work. .85
Basic Mycology Summary 87

Chapter 8   Basic Virology. 89

Part 1: Characteristics of Viruses 90
Part 2: Replication of Viruses 94
Part 3: Classification of Viruses 98
Part 4: Medically Significant Viruses 102
Part 5: How Antiviral Drugs Work 113
Basic Virology Summary 116

Chapter 9   Basic Parasitology 118

Part 1: Characteristics and Classification of Parasites . . 119
Part 2: Medically Significant Parasites and
Antiparasitic Drugs 122
Basic Parasitology Summary 128

Chapter 10   129

Bibliography. 133

FOREWORD

It gives me immense pleasure to write the foreword to the book "IT'S A SMALL WORLD AFTER ALL - Life under The Microscope" written by Mr Jesper Leonard Vun, a distinction undergraduate medical student.

When the COVID-19 pandemic started and the lockdown period began, people were getting addicted to social media. I really appreciate that my student, Jesper, made the best use of his time. Congratulations for this great effort. I am sure you will find many more books authored by Jesper.

This book gives a good insight into the world of Microbiology and it is presented so well that even the common man could understand. It takes through important information regarding bacteria, viruses, parasites and fungi. The concept of writing with 'Food for Thought' at the end is impressive.

In conclusion, it is an honour to introduce this enthusiastically written book and I salute its publication. Kudos to Mr. Jesper Vun for the great job, which has been executed well for providing basic information in simple language with illustrations in an attractive manner.

Best wishes

Dr Indira Bairy
Professor and Former Head of Microbiology
Manipal University College Malaysia (MUCM), Manipal, India

PREFACE

The whole world came to a standstill when the World Health Organization (WHO) declared the novel coronavirus, COVID-19 a pandemic. Countries after countries began closing their borders and locking down cities on an unprecedented scale in efforts to curb the spread of a contagious disease the virus brought upon humanity. Movement restrictions, curfews and quarantine orders were imposed and it undoubtedly affected millions of lives. It was a war against a force invisible to the naked eye. It was a battle fought by almost every country on the face of the earth. Those few weeks, if not months, was a period in time permanently engraved into the minds of many.

This event got me thinking, if there was ever a time the general populace needed an easily comprehensible source of information about the microscopic world, it would be now. Amidst these hard moments, many have sought information from the internet. Social media especially played a huge role in directing the thoughts and actions of people with their contents. Evidently, there were many golden nuggets that people picked up from legitimate sources but unfortunately fake news and misinformation spread much faster. It came to my notice that people tend to get a few facts right but don't quite understand the concept and significance behind it.

One day while I was explaining something regarding the virus to my parents, they suggested that I should write a book about the subject, to clear the worrisome doubts in hearts of people. I brushed off the idea at first because people could benefit more reading textbooks but later realized that it was necessary to be done. The knowledge of biology and microbiology should be made easily understandable for the common man so that with this foundation, people can realize just how much something so small can impact something big just like how a virus can even be the death of a human being. It's a given that learning something about the microscopic world today will better prepare us for the next outbreak.

I did not want my book to be a boring one with just facts and figures. Therefore, I challenged myself to make this book not only about learning microbiology but also bringing you, the reader on a journey of self-discovery and reflection so that together, we can be more appreciative of the little things, situations and circumstances we don't normally give a second thought. I got my inspiration when I stumbled across old YouTube documentaries and videos of renowned biologists and physicists that I used to watch growing up as a child. These videos were the reason I delved into the field of science. They preached the message of inquisition. I always thought that the same could inspire many more people and I bring forth the same message into my writings in this book, sharing some of my favourite quotes.

In the introduction, I give a short story about a day in the life of a businessman while sneaking in certain scenarios of how the invisible world of microbiology can influence what is visible. I thought a story like this could help you realize the relevance of microbiology even in the life of a common man. Aside from discussing the topic at hand in every chapter, I bring forth ideas as a food for thought for readers to ponder and reflect upon how the topic impacts our appreciation and outlook of life on earth. If done right, your perspective on creation would most definitely be renewed upon completion of the book.

Similar to my previous book *Medical Myth or Fact?*, I worded the descriptions in an easy to understand manner so that anyone could benefit from it. My principle remains the same, everyone is entitled to knowledge. Things should not be inaccessible just because they are hard to understand. Furthermore, I've also included personally customized visual aids such as diagrams, illustrations, flowcharts, and tables to effectively and efficiently convey information.

It was indeed a humbling experience for me in this journey of presenting this book to you and I sincerely hope that you enjoy reading and benefiting from it as much as I enjoyed writing it. Just like how small actions make a big impact, the *Micros* dictates *Macros*. In the end you will see that actually, it's a small world after all.

Jesper Leonard Vun

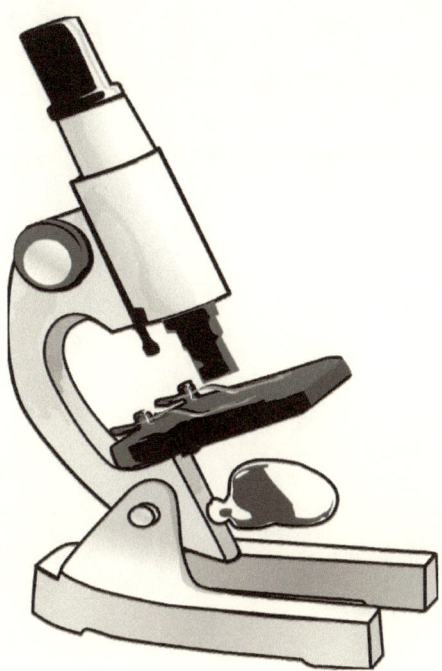

INTRODUCTION

12ᵗʰ March 2020
Thursday

Ahh...ahh...ahh...Choooooo!

I couldn't take it anymore. That was the seventh time I've sneezed since I got up five minutes ago. My nose was completely stuffed with mucus and it had been flowing down my nostrils like waterfalls. As if it wasn't already hard enough to breathe through my mouth, my throat started to itch and tingle. Not only was I trying to fight down the impulse to cough, I think I was also beginning to run a fever. *Ugh, I don't feel so good. Perhaps I should call in sick. Just for today.*

My arm was about to reach for my phone beside my bed when I remembered that I had a very important presentation to give at today's meeting. If I skipped this one, my project would never get approved by the board of directors and I will have to kiss my dream of becoming project manager goodbye. I'm not willing to let this go just because I'm having a dumb cold. Never.

I mustered every iota of strength my muscles could generate and forced myself to sit up from bed. As if on cue, a pang of pain shot through my temples. I quickly ran my fingers on it and applied pressure. I could feel the arteries pulsating on both sides. *This headache isn't going to do me any good.* I needed to get some painkillers from the drawer downstairs. I tried to stand on my feet and felt this unusual pressure build up inside my face. I gently pressed my facial bones around the nose and it hurt. From past experience, I knew my sinuses are all clogged up. My body felt sore; my muscles screamed as if it had been through war. I stretched my arms up in the air and my joints gave off this weird sensation that they haven't been used in ages.

Yup, it's official. I'm sick!

With all my might I dragged myself down the stairs towards the kitchen to get my daily dose of coffee. I stared at the clock hanging on the wall. 8.00 am. My wife would have already sent our kids to school and went to the market to get groceries. I have been pulling all-nighters for the past three days, putting together the perfect proposal that I would have to present later at 3.00p.m. in the office. Hence, my wife spared me of my household duties and allowed me to sleep in - at least, until after my meeting.

As I approached the counter top, I noticed that coffee was already prepared. It was sitting there waiting for me. A note on the kettle read:

**Gonna be back after noon. Dropping over at
Nancy's to help with her pottery.
Goodluck for your presentation! Go break a leg ;D**

I grinned. I poured myself a nice, hot cup of that aromatic concoction and went to get myself something to eat. I pulled up a loaf of bread and took a piece out. I was too lazy to get the jam so I decided I'll take it plain, just to fill up on some food before I go get the medicine. As I drew the bread closer to my mouth, I noticed a greenish hue at the opposite end of it. I instantly dropped it on the table for inspection. Just as I thought, it was mold. I checked the expiration date on the package and found that it had passed the 'best before' by three days. What a waste. I took the entire pack and disposed of it into the bin. Wouldn't want anyone getting sick taking spoiled food. I decided to munch down on some biscuits instead.

After breakfast, I made my way to the medicine drawer to find myself a paracetamol. To my dismay, we were out of it. The only thing left in there were some deworming tablets we used to take yearly. I then decided I need to see a doctor. I could drop by the clinic before I punch in for work. I'm sure it was nothing more than the common flu but figured it'll be best to get some reassurance. And medication.

I took a nice hot shower, slipped into some comfortable clothes and got in my car. I started the engine and turned on the AC. As soon as the first wave of cold air hit my face, I completely lost control. I coughed and coughed and coughed. I could feel the pressure building up behind my eyeballs. *Not good, not good.* My chest muscles ached and I could somehow feel that my diaphragm had been sucked up into my chest cavity. The tussive episode seemed to go on forever. I gave out a cry of frustration and forced down the impulse to stop the hackling torment. It took several tries before I succeeded. And in due time. Breathing was starting to get difficult. I could have sworn if I coughed a second longer my lungs would've come out.

I looked at myself in the rear-view mirror and realized my whole face was red. So were my eyes. "Okay," I muttered. "Doctor's it is."

I arrived at our family's physician clinic just as it opened. I took a deep breath and got out of the car. Upon opening the door, I immediately noticed the difference in the environment. The air smelled of disinfectant; the two nurses at the registration counter wore scrubs, hair nets, safety goggles and surgical masks. But more than that, their eyes betrayed the expression those masks were hiding underneath - the look of concern. A middle-aged woman with a child who was barely ten, both wearing face masks, was sitting at the far corner of the waiting area. My heart rate doubled at such a sight. This made my chest tighten and another tormentful bout of coughs was about to erupt. I stood dead in my tracks for a few seconds, summoning inner strength to push the urge back down my trachea. I failed.

I coughed my lungs out. My entire posture was as if I had been kneed in the stomach.

"Sir! Sir!" a voice echoed from somewhere in the background. "Are you okay?"

"Cover your mouth for God's sake!" yelled the woman from the corner as she nudged her child to move further away from me.

The nurses eventually came for my aid. One came close and patted me on the back, offering me a mask. The other went to get me a cup of water from the dispenser down the corridor. After what felt like ages, the coughing stopped and I allowed myself to take a seat. I was completely exhausted. I closed my eyes and took a sip of that lukewarm water that was soothing to the throat. Saving grace.

Beep.

My eyes opened wide. I hadn't realized that my temperature was being taken by the nurse using an infrared thermometer. "Sir, you're having a fever. 38.8°C. You need to come with us to the other room. Now."

Weakly, I obliged. A lot was going through my head. I didn't know what was going on. Why was everyone wearing personal protective equipment? Why was I being moved into an isolated room? This wasn't how we were normally treated every time my family visited Dr. Sam. I had a million more doubts but felt too weak to ask. I figured I'll soon get an explanation from the kind doctor when I meet him. I was ushered into a room at the end of the corridor, but before she closed the door behind me, I managed a peep through the narrow gap and saw that the other nurse was already disinfecting the chair I sat only barely a minute ago. She was spraying it and the atmosphere around it with an aerosol spray- no doubt some sort of disinfectant. I was utterly confused.

I hesitated sitting on the examination bed, thinking I might spare them the trouble of disinfecting it but I decided to sit anyways. My head was banging. I ransacked my brain for any possible reason so much precautionary measures were taken against a man having the common flu. Unfortunately, I couldn't find any. My mind was clouded.

"It's now a pandemic John," a familiar voice spoke, absorbing me back into the present. "They announced it yesterday."

"Who?" I asked.

"Exactly! WHO as in W-H-O, the World Health Organization," Standing right in front of me was a man dressed in full protective gear with even more layers than the nurses outside. If it weren't for that recognizable voice, no one could blame me if I guessed a madman was hiding underneath that suit. Dr. Sam and I go way back; we've been friends since high school. He sat down in front of me with his clipboard in hand. "It's getting serious John. Our area reported 3 new positive cases of the virus. And that was just yesterday! Hence, such extreme precautions. The government is working on contact tracing as we speak. So, what seems to be the problem? My nurse told me that you were coughing pretty badly out there and that you are having a fever? How long has it been going on?"

"Erm…" I started to get a little nervous at the mention of the virus outbreak. I hadn't known that W.H.O. declared it a pandemic yesterday. I was too caught up with work and it hadn't really crossed my mind. No wonder everyone was being so careful. "Actually, I've been feeling quite weak these days. Perhaps it's because I've been working late into the night. But I got up this morning sneezing and coughing like mad. That's when the fever started too. My muscles are aching and my chest feels like it's on fire."

"Any phlegm?"

"Not so far. No."

"Any travel history?"

Uh-oh. It entirely slipped my mind. At that point in time, I didn't really think it mattered so much. Plus, it was only a short two-day business trip. *He's not going to like my answer.* "I got back about two weeks ago from a business trip in Bangkok."

I could make out the frown that was forming underneath his mask. I started to panic. What were the odds that I might have contracted this new disease? I guessed my expression painted a nice picture of my concerns. Dr. Sam went on to explain that Bangkok was one of the hotspots of the virus spread. The virus was believed to be transmitted by respiratory droplets. Meaning, if someone sneezes or coughs, these droplets containing the virus could enter into another person either directly-if in close proximity, or indirectly - touching something the infected person has touched and later touching your own nose, eyes and or mouth. The incubation period, which is the time taken between the exposure to the virus and the manifestation of symptoms is about 2 to 14 days. He advised that I should go to the hospital without delay and have myself tested. I would have to isolate myself from my family and friends until the results are out. If it was unfavourable, then all my contacts since my arrival at the airport two weeks ago would have to be traced and checked for.

"Sam, you have to help me," I pleaded desperately. "I can't get this disease. Can't you just give me some antibiotic. My immune system is strong. I'm sure all I'll need is a few days of rest and then I'll be back on my feet, fit as a fiddle. Please."

"I'm sorry John," he said apologetically. "Under normal circumstances, I'll take you under my care. But given that you have such a strong history pointing towards the likelihood of having this disease, it's only the responsible thing to do to report to the hospital. For the sake of your loved ones and the community. Besides, there are currently no specific drug treatments for this virus. Antibiotics only work for bacterial infections."

"So, what about the two people outside?" I asked, ashamed of my earlier behaviour of coughing without any etiquette. "I coughed really bad in front of them."

"Don't worry about it. They were seated quite far from you and were well protected. I'll just ask them to wash their hands. Actually, they came asking for a flu vaccine. The child's mother read on WhatsApp that the vaccine can help prevent this virus. I told them it wasn't true and further clarified a few more myths. I tell you, fake news travels faster than lightning these days. As of now, you need to get to the hospital my friend. And I need to clean up your mess."

I did as the doctor ordered and rushed to the hospital. On my way, I rang up the office to call in sick and assigned my partner to take over the presentation later. I then called my wife and explained the whole story. As expected, she got really worried and angry at the same time. I just told her that it'll probably take a day for the results to come out and I would most likely be quarantined in the hospital. If all goes well then, they should be fine too; if results were not so well, then they would have to all report to the hospital tomorrow. I can't help but feel regretful over how careless I had been. I should have taken this virus outbreak more seriously and isolated myself when I came back. Now, my entire family's lives laid on the line. I failed as a husband and as a parent. And what about those people that I've come in contact with for the past few weeks? Just the number of lives I have put at stake made my stomach uneasy. *Stupid! Stupid! Stupid!*

When I got to the hospital, everything happened so fast the day went by in a blur. They took a detailed history and decided to take me in for admission into an isolated room as doctors suspected I had pneumonia. Hospital staff took a chest X-ray, a throat swab and blood samples from me for laboratory analysis and put me on an I.V. line. Multiple drugs were injected into my vein to help with my symptoms. I remained drowsy the whole day. My family were not allowed to visit so the only company I had were the beeping machines around me and the constant flow of nurses and doctors that came in to check on me every hour or so.

I was anxious to know my results. My life and those of my loved ones for the next few weeks seemed to depend on the mathematical sign of +positive or -negative. It's funny how something so small, invisible to the naked eye, can have so much impact on the lives of man, a creature at the pinnacle of evolution. Despite the fatigue, I didn't get much of a shut eye the whole night. My mind kept swirling around the uncertainties the following morning would bring and what I could have done to prevent this, for myself, my wife, and children. I had only myself to blame.

After what felt like an eternity, morning came. A doctor came into my room with some papers in hand. I didn't recognize her with all the protection on but the name tag she wore revealed her identity - Dr. Dalila. "Your results are out John."

"Give me the good news doc," I humbly requested.

She raised her gaze from the papers she was studying and looked at me. Although her face was concealed, I was certain she gave me a smile.

"COVID-19……negative."

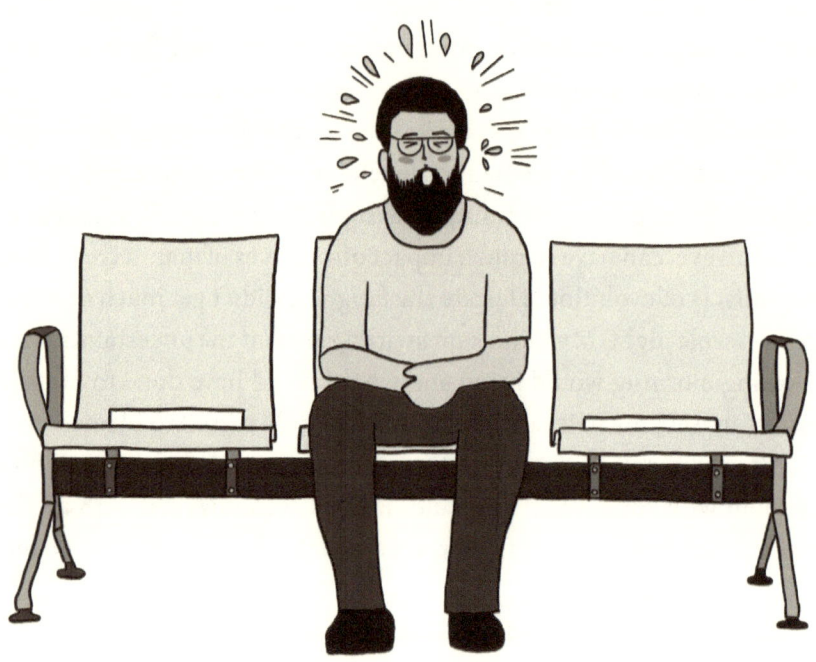

The Basic Unit of Life

Did the chicken or the egg come first?

I am certain many of us have heard this timeless question at some point of our lives. You may have even came up with a fairly logical explanation for your answer as well. Be it a rational answer or simply a joke, it is an undeniable fact that in order for all life to exist, there must first be a *cell*.

If you were to ask any student who has ever studied basic science, 'What is a cell?' the correct way to answer that would be, 'a cell is the basic unit of life.' Simple. It's already worth one mark. But hold on a second, we don't normally give it an extra thought. The basic unit of life means that without this fundamental building block, all life on earth, be it plants or animals would cease to exist. As children, we learn to differentiate between the living and the non-living. All living things are made up of cells. Though cells may not be the smallest component that goes into the pot that makes a being alive, it is however the most simple, basic, fundamental, essential and most importantly, functional unit that gives the non-living life.

And so in this chapter, we shall embark on a mission to learn about the beauty of this basic unit of life, to get a clear picture of its makeup, its components, and its function.

A microscope is a device that allows humans to see a world invisible to the naked eye. Although there is some controversy over the first person to have actually invented the microscope. The most accepted people thought to be its original inventors were Hans and Zacharias Janssen, a father and son team of spectacle makers. No matter who it may be, the first compound microscope became the stepping stone for the more powerful ones we have today. The electron microscope for example. Since its invention in the late sixteenth century by the Dutch duo, a whole new branch of study was developed — Microbiology.

Microbiology is the scientific study of microorganisms, which paved the way to the revolutionary things we have understood and accomplished in a world we cannot see. For starters, the ideal specimens to view under the microscope would be cells from the scrapings of the inside of the human cheek (cheek cells), and the thin layer peeled from the inside of an onion (plant cells). This is just to get a glimpse of what an animal cell (cheek cell) and a plant cell look like. If you were to peer through the lenses of the compound light microscope, you would be able to observe hundreds of circular or oval shaped structures with a central black dot. These are cells. In the case of plant cells, they would be stacked in a regular pattern, which is really hard to miss.

If we were to single the cells out individually, they would look something like this:

Animal cells (cheek cells):

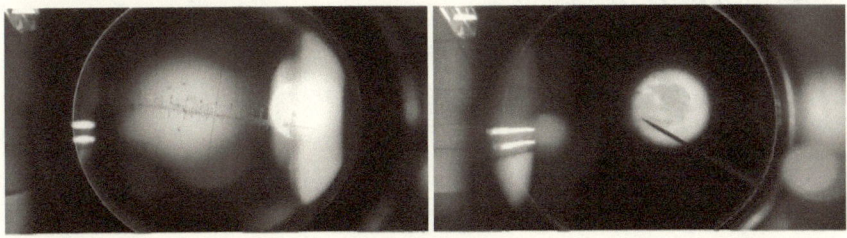

Plant cells of an onion:

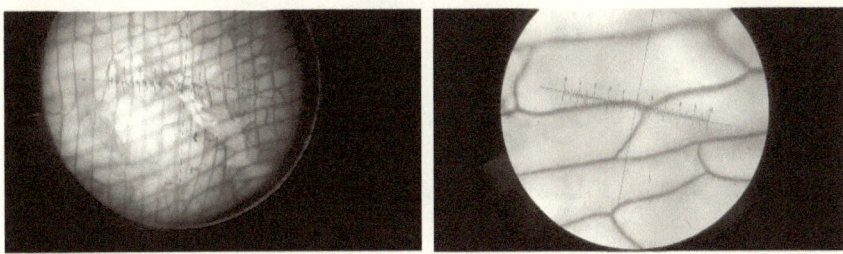

However, cells are much more than what you would be able to see from just a compound light microscope. If we were to use a stronger and more powerful microscope, like the electron microscope, then we could view these cells in stunning detail. The tiny dots scattered within the cytoplasm of the cell are called *organelles* — small organs. Just like any larger life forms, cells require the functioning of smaller organs to make them whole and alive. And these organelles take up different shapes and sizes.

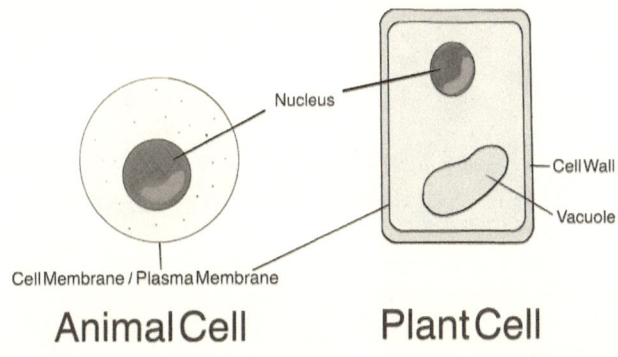

We are going to dive deeper into the structures along with their function(s) that make a cell.

COMPONENT	DESCRIPTION &FUNCTION
Nucleus:	• Membrane bounded organelle • Largest organelle • Stores genetic information (e.g. DNA-deoxyribonucleic acid) which codes for protein *synthesis* • Controls all cellular activity
Cytoplasm:	• A jelly-like medium where all the organelles of the cell are located • Many biochemical processes of the cell take place in the cytoplasm
Plasma membrane:	• Membrane consisting of two layers made of phospholipids • a.k.a. phospholipid bilayer • Contains protein and other molecules like cholesterol • Separates the external environment from the internal environment of the cell • Acts as a semi permeable membrane and allows transport of substance in and out of the cell

Cell wall: 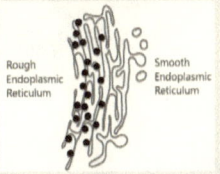	• Found in plant cells and many species of bacteria and fungi • Surrounds the plasma membrane • Provides mechanical as well as structural support to the cell
Endoplasmic reticulum: 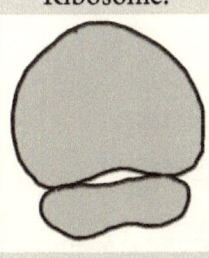	Smooth endoplasmic reticulum: • Synthesizes steroids • Detoxifies drugs and poisons Rough endoplasmic reticulum: • Synthesizes secretory proteins (for export out of cell)
Ribosome: 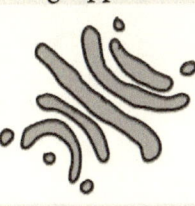	• Made of two subunits. • Site of protein synthesis
Golgi apparatus:	• Modifies, transports, sorts and packages protein

Lysosome:

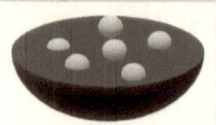

- Membrane bounded organelle
- A small sac containing digestive enzymes (hydrolytic enzymes)
- Acts as the digestive compartment of the cell

Peroxisome:

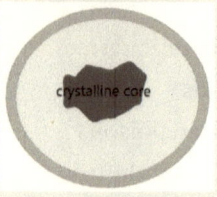

- Membrane bounded organelle
- Breaks down chains of fatty acid
- Detoxifies hydrogen peroxide and other harmful compounds

Centrioles:

- Forms spindle fibers during cell division
- Not found in plant cells

Cytoskeleton

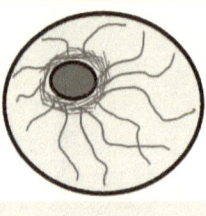

Cell

- Consist of microfilaments, intermediate filaments and microtubules
- Supports the shape and movement of the cell

Mitochondria:

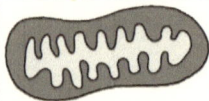

- Double membrane bounded
- Powerhouse of the cell
- Site of *cellular respiration* — releases energy for the cell through the breakdown of food substances
- Contains its own set of DNA passed down only from the maternal line

Chloroplast: 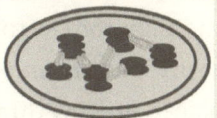	• Double membrane bounded • Contains green pigments called chlorophyll • Site of *photosynthesis*
Vacuole: 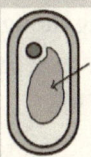	• Fluid filled sac with a semi-permeable membrane • Storage site of the cell

Synthesis: To produce

Cellular respiration: A set of biochemical reactions that takes place in the cell to convert nutrients into energy that can be used readily by the cell in the form of ATP (Adenosine triphosphate) and releasing waste products.

Photosynthesis: The process where green plants and certain fungi and bacteria uses light energy from the sun to synthesize nutrients from carbon dioxide and water, generating oxygen as a by-product.

It is important that we familiarize ourselves with the components and structure of the common animal cell and plant cell as it is imperative to understand the differences between the two different cell types: *prokaryotic cells* and *eukaryotic cells* which will be discussed in further chapters.

We now come to the question: How does a single cell make us whole?

Life, as we know it today, began from a single cell. As the world renowned English broadcaster and natural historian, Sir David Attenborough puts it, *'All life is related, and it enables us to construct with confidence, the complex tree that represents the history of life.'*

In his documentary entitled, 'Charles Darwin and the Tree of Life,' he described that all life began in the sea where complex molecules grouped into a cluster that formed a cell. This was the seed that gave rise to the tree of life. As time passed, the tree of life diversified to give rise to all the different organisms on earth that we see today. From a cell in the sea, these pioneering organisms evolved over time to conquer land.

You may want to take some time to appreciate and allow the fact to sink in that our planet Earth, is, as far as we know, unique in the entire universe. It is the only planet that contains life. This lonely planet, drifting through the void of space and time harbours such a number of different plants and animal species that even we, in the entire course of human history, have not even named all of them. It's indeed a fascinating thought that all life, though different in shapes and sizes, can be traced back through an unbroken thread to the same ancestral cell. The seed of life.

From unicellular organisms such as the bacteria and protozoans to more complex multicellular organisms like the fungi, plants, and animals, this can only be achieved through *differentiation* and *specialization* of cells. This is how a human, a body of 37.2 trillion cells, each with its own specific function stem from a single cell (the fertilized ovum).

Cellular differentiation and specialization are the processes by which a stem cell (a cell capable of unlimited cell division and becoming any specialized cell; a generic cell) transforms/differentiates into a specific cell that carries out a specific function. For example, stem cells in the bone marrow can differentiate into red blood cells (RBCs) that carry oxygen or into white blood cells (WBCs) that help fend off infections by invading microorganisms.

Cell: The basic structural and functional unit of life (e.g. RBC)

Tissue: A group of similar cells with the same function to carry out a particular job (e.g. blood)

Organ: A group of different tissues performing a specific function (e.g. heart)

System: A group of different organs working together to do a particular job (e.g. cardiovascular system)

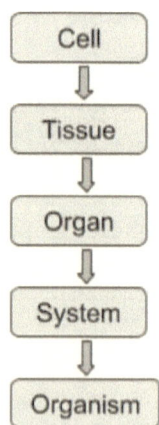

Cellular Hierarchy

This kind of cell organization is necessary as it allows a multicellular organism like us to:

1. Efficiently perform a specific task
2. Perform a variety of tasks and function in an orderly fashion through the division of work among cells
3. Attain a higher growth rate
4. Adapt and thrive in diverse living environment

To sum up this chapter, all living things are made of tiny building blocks of life called cells. Cells contain *organelles* that help them carry out essential functions of life. Living things can be either *unicellular* or *multicellular*. Multicellular organisms have cells that *differentiate, specialize,* and form a *hierarchy* to carry out specific functions for survival.

FOOD FOR THOUGHT:

What are the odds that Earth may be the only place in the entire universe where the environment is conducive enough that chemicals clump together to give rise to the seed of life from which you and I both stem from? Are we, together with everything else that breaths, an accident of that fateful event, or was it all by design? Think about it. That's the beauty.

CHAPTER 2

The Body's Defences

When we think about small beings, cuteness is usually the first impression most people will get. Babies, puppies, kittens, even a tiger' or lion's cub are cute. Unfortunately, when we scrutinize the world under the microscope, cute and cuddly is the last thing many will expect to find. Some species may be harmless, but a significant number of them are ever ready to cause you a great deal of harm, if not kill you.

However, you need not worry about them too quickly. Just like how any sovereign nation has its own standing military power to protect itself, our bodies are not left defenceless. If anything, millions of years of evolution has equipped us with impressive ways to protect ourselves and fight off these microbial invaders. An entire branch of scientific study called *immunology* was developed, dedicated to learn about the ways our body defends itself so that this knowledge can be used for the greater good of boosting human immunity and maybe even using it to fight cancer. It's no stroll in the park. Hence, this chapter simplifies the basics we should know about the human body's defences — the *immune system*.

In general, our immune system has three lines of defence.

1. **First line of defence:** Physical and/or chemical barriers (natural barriers)
2. **Second line of defence:** Non-specific immune response
3. **Third line of defence:** Specific immune response

Another way we could categorize this is as follows:

1. **Innate immunity:** includes first and second lines of defence (these are non-specific)
2. **Acquired/adaptive immunity:** includes the third line of defence (this is specific)

We will deal with each one of them in further detail.

First line of defence

- The first line of defence comprises the natural barriers of the body that restricts the entry of microorganisms. E.g. skin and mucous membranes.
- It is non-specific. Meaning, it does not discriminate microbes that are harmless from those that actually do damage. It will block out any of them.
- All portals of entry are guarded with this line of defence using various mechanisms.

PORTAL OF ENTRY	MECHANISM OF DEFENCE
Skin	• Forms a physical barrier to prevent microorganisms from entering the body • Has a dry, dead, proteinaceous layer called the keratin layer that forms this blockade • Oily secretions (sebum) from sebaceous glands in the skin provides a protective film on the skin and prevents microbial growth; has antimicrobial properties
Nose	• Nostrils have hair to minimize entry of fine particles • Antibodies (IgA) lines the mucous membrane to prevent attachment of invading microorganism • Trachea is lined by cells with cilia (finger-like projections) that sweeps foreign particles up and away from the lungs • Cough reflex / Sneeze reflex to clear the respiratory tract of any foreign particles
Mouth	• Saliva has antimicrobial properties
Ears	• Ear wax (cerumen) to trap foreign particles and prevent entry of microbes
Eyes	• Tears has antimicrobial properties
Urogenital Tract	• Flushing mechanism during micturition (urination) • Vagina has an acidic pH to prevent growth of *pathogenic* microorganism

Pathogenic; pathogen: Microorganisms that causes harm/damage to the human body

It should be noted that these portals of entry as well as other parts of the body such as parts of the digestive tract naturally harbour harmless microorganisms. Chiefly, bacteria. They are called *normal flora.* In a healthy individual, normal floras do not pose as a threat but rather, they provide a person with various benefits:

- They compete with pathogen for nutrients so that they cannot thrive
- In the gut, normal flora synthesizes vitamin K
- They stimulate production of antibodies
- They maintain an acidic environment in the vagina to prevent infection

However, there are also downsides to having normal floras. Though generally harmless, they may cause opportunistic infections when there is a breach in the first line defences. For example, a cut injury on the skin will allow the access of all sorts of microorganisms into the body. Certain species will seize this opportunity to invade the body and cause harm. Hence the term, opportunistic.

A breach in the first line of defence will activate the second line of defence.

Second line of defence

In order to understand this line of defence, it is important to first grasp the basics about blood.

To most of us, blood is just the red fluid that bleeds out of the wound whenever we are injured or when healthcare personnel draw them out for analysis. We know that it's vital for life; we know that it carries oxygen to all parts of the body and not enough of it will cause death. Otherwise, we don't give it much thought. Well, this fluid of life is actually not as simple as it may seem. It holds secrets; it holds information; it holds identity; it holds indications; it gives protection; it's a mode of transport for chemicals and proteins. Here's a comprehensible breakdown of blood.

Blood is a collective term for several components. Ever wonder what happens to your blood outside the body? Why is it that blood clots and hardens after a while whenever we sustain a wound injury but when doctors draw it out of our veins, it remains in a fluid state? Simple. The containers (vacutainers) where blood is stored are lined with agents that prevent it from clotting. The blood samples are then put into a machine (centrifuge) and spun around really quickly, allowing the blood components to segregate and sedimentate. The final product shows three separate layers: plasma, buffy coat and red blood cells. Plasma (~55%) contains water, proteins, nutrients, ions, wastes and gases. The buffy coat (~1%) represents the white blood cells and platelets.

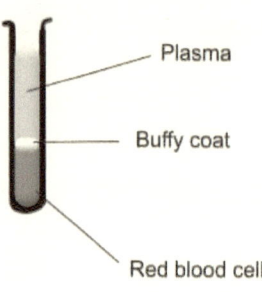

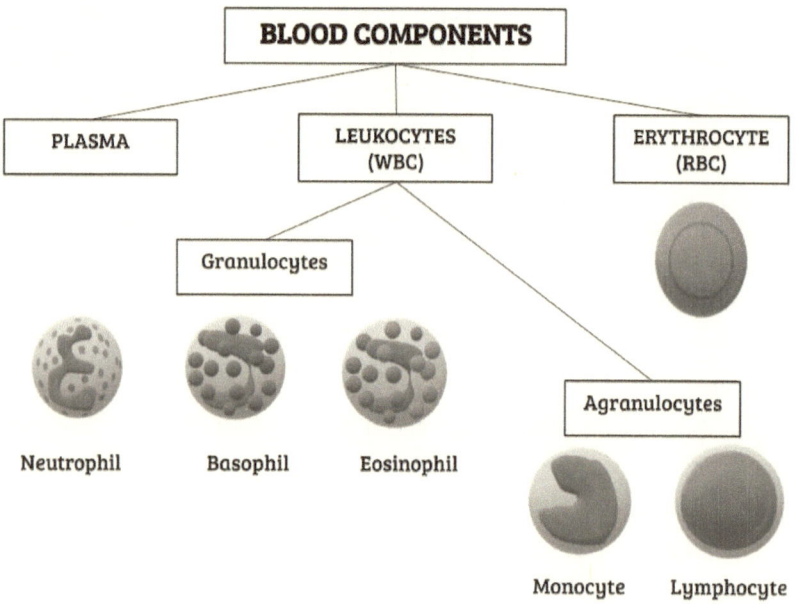

Cytes- cells; *leuko*- white; *erythro*- red

With regards to our body's defences, we are more focused on the WBC/leukocytic component of blood. The number of WBCs is about 4000-11000 cells/mm^3 of blood.

Granulocytes:

They are known as granulocytes because these cells contain granules of enzymes that help in the digestion/killing of pathogens.

GRANULOCYTE	DESCRIPTION/FUNCTIONS
Neutrophil:	• Multi-lobed nucleus • Contains granules • Kills invading microbes by *phagocytosis* • Normal range: 50%-70%
Eosinophil:	• Bi-lobed/double lobed nucleus • Contains granules (red in colour) • Involved in allergic reactions and parasitic infection • Normal range: 1%-4%
Basophil:	• Bi-lobed/ double lobed nucleus • Contains granules (dark blue in colour) • Involved in allergic reactions • Normal range: 0%-1%

Agranulocytes:

These cells *do not* contain granules. Hence the name agranulocyte. The prefix 'a-' indicates the absence of-.

AGRANULOCYTE	DESCRIPTION/FUNCTIONS
Monocytes:	• Kidney shaped nucleus • Differentiates into macrophages • Found in the blood • Normal range: 2%-8%
Macrophages;	• Differentiated from monocytes • Found in body tissues • Kill invading microbes by *phagocytosis*
Lymphocytes:	• Large nucleus, scanty cytoplasm • Consists of two types: T cell and B cell • Not involved in innate immunity/ first and second line of defence • Involved in *adaptive immunity* (described later) • Normal range: 20%-40%

Phagocytosis: Cell eating by extending its false feet/ pseudopodia and enveloping the microbe, which later forms a phagosome that fuses with the lysosome for digestion.

Process of phagocytosis:

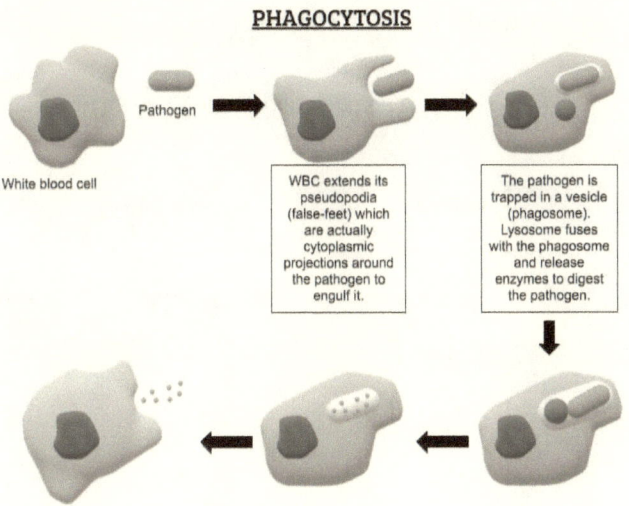

PHAGOCYTOSIS

Pathogen

White blood cell

WBC extends its pseudopodia (false-feet) which are actually cytoplasmic projections around the pathogen to engulf it.

The pathogen is trapped in a vesicle (phagosome). Lysosome fuses with the phagosome and release enzymes to digest the pathogen.

All the above-mentioned leukocytes except the agranular lymphocytes are involved in the second line of defence, a non-specific immune response.

These cells do not discriminate against any species of invading microorganism, be it a bacterium that causes pneumonia; a fungus that causes aspergillus; or even a parasite that causes diarrhoea, as long as it's foreign to the body, they will respond.

Third line of defence

Also known as the *adaptive/acquired immunity*
Here, lymphocytes take the spotlight.
As mentioned, there are two types of lymphocytes:

1. T cells
2. B cells

T cells can be further subdivided into *killer (cytotoxic) T cells, helper T cells, suppressor T cells* and *memory T cells.* They constitute the *cell-mediated immunity.*

B cells on the other hand are capable of differentiating into *plasma cells* which are capable of forming antibodies. B cells also form *memory B cells*. They constitute the *humoral immunity*.

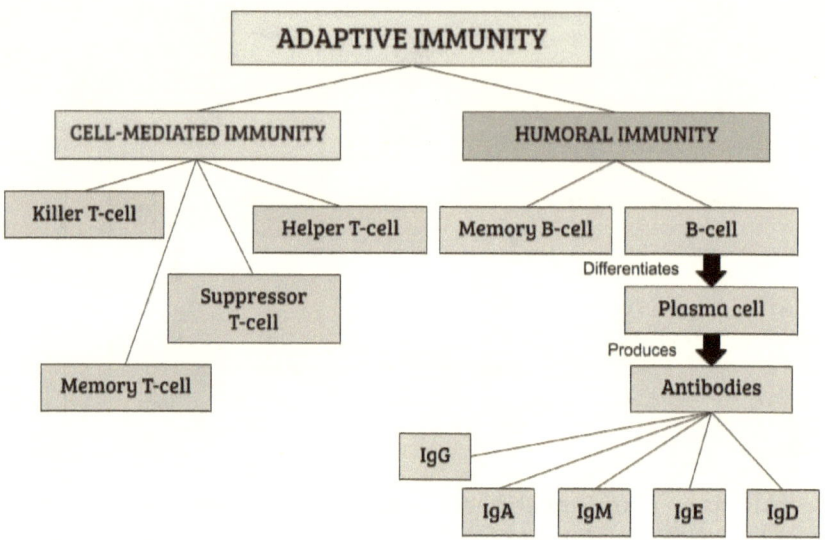

There are five different types of antibodies (immunoglobulins):

TYPE	DESCRIPTION/FUNCTION
IgM	• First antibody to arise during an infection (takes approximately 5-7 days to form)
IgG	• Arises later than IgM • The only antibody that can cross the placenta to provide immunity to the developing fetus

IgA	• Found on mucous membranes. Otherwise known as *secretory antibody* • Prevents attachment of pathogens onto mucus membranes • Found in colostrum (first breast milk). Hence it is advisable to breastfeed newborns.
IgE	• Involved in allergic reactions and parasitic infections
IgD	• Found on the surface of B cells • Act as receptors for antigens to signal B cell activation

The adaptive immunity is characterized as follows:

- **A highly specific immune response**

  Unlike the innate immunity, adaptive immunity is mounted specifically towards one particular pathogen. It is ineffective against another.

- **Having a lag period**

  A varying period of time (days to weeks) is needed before acquired immunity can mount a response towards the pathogen. This differs from innate immunity, which is ever present and ever ready.

- **Produces memory cells**

  After recovery, the person develops memory cells so that a second or subsequent exposure to the same pathogen will result in a more rapid and efficient immune response (shorter lag period).

Innate immunity does not 'remember'. Mainly because they have no need to. They are indiscriminate in their killing.

- **Has a longer lasting immunity**

Immunity towards a specific pathogen can last for years. Some, even decades.

Here's an example to paint you a clearer picture:

Six-year-old Katie was waiting in line to go down the slide on the playground when the boy in front of her turned around and sneezed. The respiratory droplets containing the measles virus enter her nostrils. The virus managed to bypass her first and second line of defences. About a week later, she fell ill and developed a cough, fever and red eyes (conjunctivitis). After three days, she started seeing rashes all over her body. She continued to have these symptoms for six days *(the lag period)* before it faded away. Little did she know that the lymphocytes in her have been activated and are at war with the virus. T cells started killing virus infected cells and B cells were producing antibodies to neutralize the virus. These lymphocytes did nothing more than kill the measles virus *(specific immune response)*. She began to feel better. On the fourteenth day, she fully recovered. The T and B cells then formed *memory cells*. Unbeknownst to Katie, she again caught the same measles virus two years later while she was playing with her friends but she never developed the disease again *(long lasting immunity)*. This is because her memory T and B cells proliferated rapidly and efficiently to kill off the virus.

If Katie were to be infected by a different type of virus, for example the mumps virus, the immunity against the measles virus would be useless against it due to the *specificity* of the adaptive immunity. She would have to go through the entire process of building up this immunity again for the new virus.

To summarize: the human immune systems consist of three lines of defence. The first and second lines mount non-specific responses and are categorized as innate immunity. The third line of defence mounts a specific immune response. It is also called adaptive/acquired immunity. The first line of defence is by natural physical and chemical barriers. The second line is protected by granulocytes, monocytes and macrophages. The third line is taken care of by the cell-mediated immunity (T cells) and humoral immunity (B cells).

FOOD FOR THOUGHT:

Isn't it wonderful that our bodies are gifted with such an amazing system of defence, without which we would have succumbed to the invisible forces of the microscopic world even at the early stages of life. Hence, it is paramount that we take good care of our health and not simply destroy it with unvirtuous activities. Once it's gone, it's gone for good. People tend to not appreciate the simple things in life until they are deprived of it. Health should not be taken for granted.

CHAPTER 3

A Vaccine in Time Saves Nine

I n the year 1796, an English doctor by the name of Edward Jenner tested the world's first vaccine for smallpox. Back then, smallpox was a highly contagious and dangerous disease caused by the smallpox virus. Its disfiguring effects affected people for thousands of years and claimed millions of lives. While Jenner was still a medical student, he realized that milkmaids who contracted cowpox, a comparatively mild blister forming disease, never contracted smallpox. On May 14 that fateful year, he took the cowpox blister fluid and inoculated it into a small eight-year-old boy. He developed the disease but recovered shortly after. Two months down the line, Jenner inoculated smallpox into the same boy but this time, he did not develop the disease. This showed that the vaccine was an epic success and it changed the course of medicine for all of mankind. Since its discovery, the smallpox vaccine has saved an estimated five million lives a year, that would bring us up to having prevented the death of about two hundred million people till date.

Today, smallpox has been declared eradicated from the face of the earth thanks to global initiatives of vaccination programmes. The next disease on its way to worldwide eradication is polio.

Vaccines are undeniably miracle drugs and many types of it have been developed over the century to prevent all sorts of diseases. As a matter of fact, newborns are immediately given vaccinations after birth and follow a strict schedule mandated by governments all over the world. No, vaccines are not a scheme for pharmaceutical companies to profit off the general public. In contrast to that, many of the mandatory ones are provided for free by the government. Why are world administrators taking vaccines so seriously? To the extent that children cannot enrol for school or adults being rejected employment just because they missed the dose.

Contrary to general beliefs, vaccines are technically not medications that are injected into the body to prevent and relieve an individual of a certain disease. It's not like injecting a person with analgesics to relieve pain. It's also not as if having been vaccinated will guarantee you will never get the disease. To put it briefly, the content of a vaccine is the disease-causing agent itself. It is introduced into the body so that adaptive immunity can be built up against it. When the person actually contracts the disease in a later time, the body would already have memory cells that can activate a more rapid and efficient immune response. The actual disease, if one ever catches it, will have much milder symptoms than it would originally have caused. Now before worrying about deliberately injecting yourself with a deadly pathogen, consider the following.

There are four different types of vaccines:

TYPE	DESCRIPTION	EXAMPLE
Live attenuated	• Contains the weakened form of the disease-causing agent • Provides a long-lasting immunity (usually lifetime with one or two doses) as it resembles the natural infection • May not be suitable for immunocompromised state • Needs refrigeration • Very rarely, viral vaccines like OPV may have the risk of the virus returning to virulent form (reversion to virulence). In simple terms, it means that the virus reverts back to its pre-weakened state and cause the disease.	• MMR (measles, mumps, rubella) • Rotavirus • Chickenpox • Yellow fever • Smallpox • Polio (OPV)-oral

Inactivated	• Contains the killed form of the disease-causing agent • Immunity doesn't last long and requires frequent booster doses	• Hepatitis A • Influenza • Rabies • Polio (IPV)-injectable
Subunit, recombinant, polysaccharide & conjugate vaccines	• Contains specific pieces of the disease-causing agent • Provides a strong immunity against the disease • Booster shots required • Suitable for most of the general populace, including the immunocompromised	• Pneumococcal disease • Meningococcal disease • Hib (Haemophilus influenzae type b) • Hepatitis B
Toxoid	• Contains the toxin that is produced by the bacteria to stimulate the production of antibodies against the toxin (not the agent)	• Tetanus • Diphtheria

Vaccines can be introduced into the body via several routes. For example, oral, intranasal (up the nostril), intradermal (within the skin), subcutaneous (below skin; above muscle) and intramuscular (within the muscle). Each vaccine has a specific route to administer accordingly.

Brief overview of the mechanism of vaccines with relation to the body's immunity.

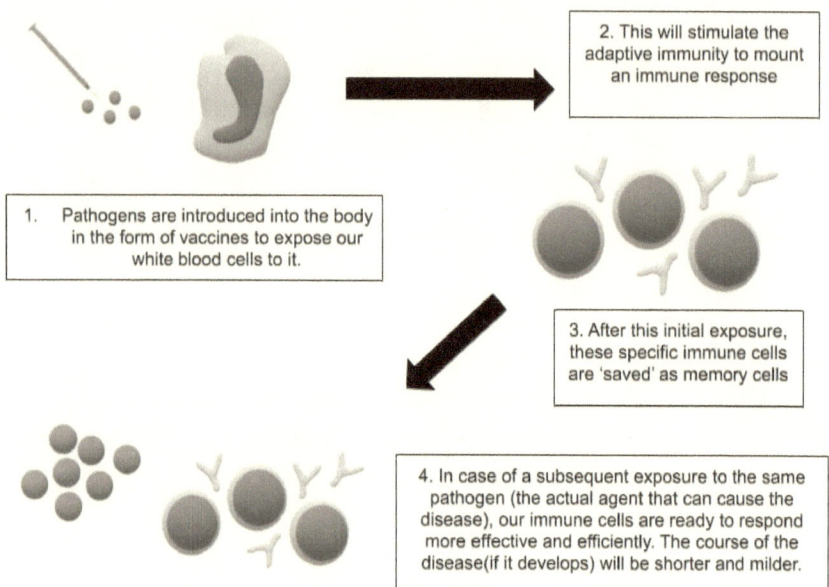

1. Pathogens are introduced into the body in the form of vaccines to expose our white blood cells to it.

2. This will stimulate the adaptive immunity to mount an immune response

3. After this initial exposure, these specific immune cells are 'saved' as memory cells

4. In case of a subsequent exposure to the same pathogen (the actual agent that can cause the disease), our immune cells are ready to respond more effective and efficiently. The course of the disease(if it develops) will be shorter and milder.

When discussing on the topic of vaccines, we cannot run far from the subject of immunity. Both come hand in hand. Immunity towards a pathogen can be acquired either *actively* or *passively*. In this context, *active* means that the body actively produces its own immunity whereas *passive* means that the body just passively receives externally made immunity.

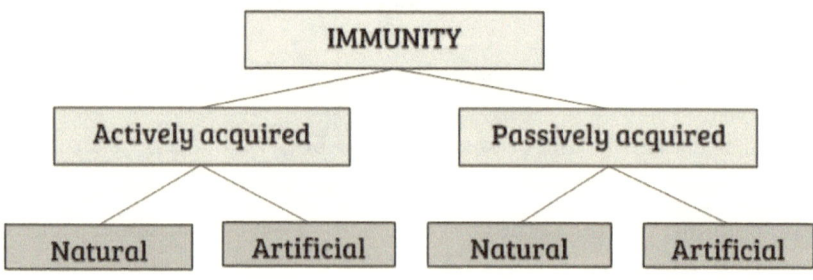

TYPES OF IMMUNITY	DESCRIPTION/EXAMPLE
Naturally acquired active immunity	• Immunity acquired following a primary (first time) infection by a pathogen where an immune response is mounted.
Artificially acquired active immunity	• Immunity acquired through vaccination (not infection)
Naturally acquired passive immunity	• Antibodies (IgG) from the mother's blood cross the placenta into the foetus to provide immunity during intrauterine life. • Antibodies (IgA) found in the colostrum of breast milk is given to infants during breastfeeding
Artificially acquired passive immunity	• Immunity acquired by receiving an injected specific antibody against a disease. • E.g. injecting tetanus immunoglobulins as management for dirty and deep wounds to prevent tetanus; injecting antivenom after a snakebite • Gives an immediate but temporary protection to the patient

The immunization schedule set by the Malaysian Ministry of Health (MoH).

AGE	TYPE OF IMMUNISATION
At birth	BCG dose 1; Hepatitis B dose 1
1 month	Hepatitis B dose 2
2 months	DTAP dose 1; Hib dose 1; Polio (IPV) dose 1
3 months	DTaP dose 2; Hib dose 2; Polio (IPV) dose 2
5 months	DTaP dose 3; Hib dose 3; Polio (IPV) dose 3
6 months	Hepatitis B dose 3; Measles dose 1 (Sabah only)
9 months	MMR dose 1; JE dose 1 (Sarawak only)
12 months	MMR dose 2
18 months	DTaP booster; Hib booster; Polio (IPV) booster
21 months	JE dose 2 (Sarawak only)
7 years	MR; DT
13 years	HPV dose 1&2
15 years	Tetanus booster

BCG: Bacillus Calmette- Guerin (for extrapulmonary tuberculosis); DTAP; Diphtheria, Tetanus & acellular Pertussis; MMR: Measles, Mumps & Rubella; JE: Japanese Encephalitis; DT: Diphtheria & Tetanus; HPV: Human Papillomavirus.

(Source: Portal Rasmi MyHealth Kementerian Kesihatan Malaysia, 27 November 2020)

To wrap it all up, vaccines save millions of lives each and every year. They work by introducing either live attenuated, inactivated, subunits or toxoid of a particular pathogen into the body to stimulate an immune response so that in the event the real disease is contracted, the body will be able to carry out a secondary response more rapidly and efficiently to rid the disease and its undesired symptoms.

FOOD FOR THOUGHT:

The importance of vaccines is unparalleled in preventing life threatening diseases. They are not drugs that cause harm, they are not some scheme by governments and pharmaceutical companies to gain big bucks, they are here for the sake of helping us survive. The threat of preventable diseases is very real! People used to die from common diseases like chickenpox, tetanus, rabies, typhoid fever, hepatitis, mumps, measles, diphtheria and more. Life expectancy of humans has increased tremendously because of these miraculous vaccines. Anti-vaxxers, a community of non-believers of vaccines, has recently gained popularity by consistently finding ways of criticizing vaccination programmes. This has become a very serious global issue as preventable diseases can creep its way back into the community and kill innocent lives because of the carelessness and hesitancy of the few. If the world can go into lockdown because of the lack of a COVID-19 vaccine, imagine how much worse it will be if people do not take vaccines that are readily available now? Do not be afraid to get vaccinated, a single dose may be the difference between life and death.

ABOUT THE COVID-19 VACCINE:

According to the CDC (Center for Disease Control and Prevention) website, there are three main types of COVID-19 vaccines.

1. mRNA vaccines

It's a genetic material which codes for the viral protein. Our own cells then use this instruction to produce these harmless proteins. After they are made, the mRNA from the vaccine is destroyed. Our own immunity recognizes that these proteins are foreign. Thus, it mounts an immune response. Memory cells are formed to protect us from the real virus in the future.

2. Protein subunit vaccines

Here, harmless COVID-19 viral proteins are used.

3. Vector vaccines

This uses a weakened version of a live virus (not COVID -19) as a vector that carries the genetic material of a COVID-19 virus. This viral vector will enter our cells and give instructions on manufacturing a protein unique to COVID-19. Once these proteins are made, our immunity will mount a response.

*These vaccines will NOT give you COVID-19.

For more information, visit the CDC website at: https://www.cdc.gov/coronavirus/2019-ncov/vaccines/different-vaccines/how-they-work.html

CHAPTER 4

A Place for Everything, Everything in its Place

Being human, we have a natural tendency to classify things. We like to create order out of the chaotic mess we live in. It is analogous to how some people couldn't bear the sight of seeing their household in a mess and will then reorganize the place so that each clothe, equipment, furniture, utensil, and electronic device has a designated place to be kept so that when needed, it could be retrieved with ease. This tendency embedded in the very nature of our being extends beyond the household. If you have ever stepped foot into a forest, you will most likely have realized the vast biodiversity that calls it home, from the smallest ant to the tallest tree. Humans being humans, some of us just can't stand the thought that everything we see on this Earth be in such a disarray and in an unorganized fashion. We like order. Hence, scientists have for centuries seen the need to formulate special organizational systems to classify the natural world that we live in so that everything has its place.

We are able to recognize patterns and similar traits in certain groups of living things that we classify them under the same category, starting from the most obvious observable trait to the least. Thus, *taxonomy* was born - an entire branch of scientific study that names, defines and classifies organisms based on shared characteristics.

The scientific nomenclature (naming) of an organism follows the below hierarchy.

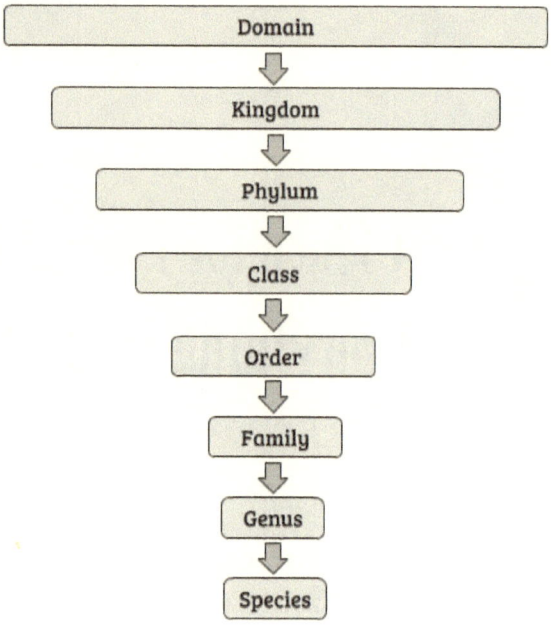

Generally, there are three domains and five kingdoms from which all life are categorized.

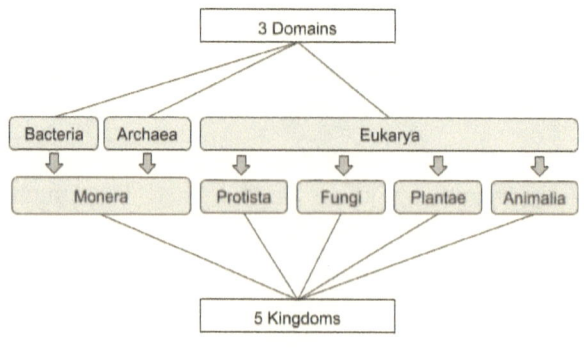

For instance, you may already know that the scientific name of humans is *Homo sapiens*. But have you ever wondered why are we called so? As a matter of fact, it's because of the long line down of taxonomy.

CATEGORY	EXAMPLE
Domain	Eukaryota
Kingdom	Animalia
Phylum	Chordata
Class	Mamalia
Order	Primates
Family	Hominidae
Genus	*Homo*
Species	*sapiens*

The scientific name of any organism is given as *Genus species*. This is called the binomial (two names) nomenclature. Hence, *Homo sapiens*. Please note that the name for genus and species are written in an Italicized manner where the first letter of the genus is capitalized but the first letter of the species is in lower case. This is a scientific standard used worldwide. Likewise, it can also be written as <u>Homo sapiens</u>.

Humans are a simple example because we are a single species. Every human across the globe is the same. We are unique in the sense that there are no other kinds like us. When we say human, we immediately imagine a being in our own image. But the need for taxonomy comes in handy when we try to describe other species. Can you imagine what it'll be like if scientists wanted to refer to an animal by giving a vague name with some description. Try picturing bird watchers without the knowledge of taxonomy. The situation would probably be something like this:

Ming: Hey John, I saw a beautiful kingfisher the other day when I went bird watching.

John: Really? Which is it?

Ming: It was blue with short tail feathers and a short beak.

John: Oh! Is it those common ones we usually see around the lake?

Ming: No, doesn't look like it. This one is different.

John: Huh, I can only picture the ones we normally see. Most kingfishers look the same if you ask me.

Unfortunately, that's as far as the conversation would have probably gone without taxonomy. If Ming could have identified that bird as *Todiramphus macleayii* (forest kingfisher) from *Alcedo atthis* (common kingfisher) -both blue in colour with short tail feathers- then the two bird enthusiasts' conversation could have lasted longer with more exchange of information.

It most definitely will take some time getting familiar with the scientific names of animals and plants that we are so used to calling cats, dogs, grass and bushes. Thankfully, there is no necessity to memorize all of them. The internet is always at our disposal. The main objective of this chapter is to make you realize the existence as well as the importance of this system of nomenclature because this knowledge will aid you deeply in the chapters to come as well as your daily life. In addition, taxonomy can help us trace the genetic relationship between species so as to connect the dots of our ancestry and the origin of life. As Jane Goodall puts it, *'There isn't a sharp line dividing us humans from the rest of the animal kingdom but it's a very woozy line and it's getting woozier all the time.'*

When we peer through the microscope onto a specimen, take a drop of water from the lake for example, you will immediately notice an abundance of tiny organisms of different shapes and sizes, twisting, turning, darting, swimming, moving or even staying still. Chaotic. Just like nature. And until we can isolate and identify every single one of them and put them into groups, nothing makes sense.

With that, we can broadly classify the microscopic world into:

1. Bacteria
2. Archaea
3. Algae
4. Fungi
5. Viruses
6. Protozoa
7. Multicellular animal parasites

For your convenience in better comprehension, some of the above topics will be merged into the same chapter due to their similarities. Details will be further discussed later in the book.

To put things shortly, we can classify all living creatures into its common category. It gets more specific down the hierarchy. This branch of study is known as taxonomy. It helps us understand a group of organisms with similar characteristics more effectively and efficiently.

FOOD FOR THOUGHT:

Carl Linnaeus was a Swedish man who lived in the eighteenth century. He is known as the father of taxonomy. From an early age, he developed a keen interest and passion for studying plants from his father's garden. He expanded his hobby and went on expeditions to classify plants and living beings. During his time, nomenclature and categorization of the natural world wasn't anything new but it was flawed. There was no common standard practiced worldwide and names were changed at will. It was his brand of classification that quickly caught wind. The system he developed is still in use today and has influenced many biologists of his time and beyond. His motivation was something of divinity. Being a son to a Lutheran pastor, he rationalized that by studying nature, it could bring man one step closer into unveiling the glory of God in the Order of His creation. Whether you believe in a divine creator or not, there is something to be taken away from his inspiration. Think of it this way, if humans are as far as we know the only living being with the highest intellectual ability in the entire universe, then we, humans, a four limbed fragile creature drifting through space on a ball of dirt and water are by far the only means for the universe to understand itself. What we understand is how much the universe understands itself. Because, if we are indeed alone, then we are at the brink of knowledge. But there is so much to be learnt. To be alive and human is an honourable and humbling experience. That's why curiosity is key. Never stop questioning. You never know how your inquiries will change the world and the course of your field. In the words of Carl Sagan, a world renowned astrophysicist, *'We are ways for the cosmos to know itself.'*

CHAPTER 5

An Introduction to Infection

In order to proceed further in discussions about various species of microorganisms, there are certain terminologies that we need to familiarize ourselves with to better understand the topics. This chapter will mainly be about defining terms that you will come across very often from henceforth.

WHAT IS AN INFECTION?

An infection is defined as the invasion and multiplication of a disease-causing agent (pathogen) in or on the tissue of a host. It should be noted that not all infections will result in a disease. Diseases are a rare consequence of infections. A disease, simply put is an abnormality that negatively impacts the structure and function of all or parts of a living thing. Diseases are not the result of immediate physical injury. They often manifest as unpleasant symptoms.

TYPES OF INFECTION:

1. Primary infection: First or initial infection
2. Re-infection: A subsequent infection by the same pathogen
3. Secondary infection: A new infection of a different pathogen on a host whose immunity has been compromised by a previous or current infection
4. Nosocomial infection: a.k.a. Hospital acquired infection
5. Endogenous infection: Source of infection is within the body
6. Exogenous infection: Source of infection is outside the body

WHAT IS A PANDEMIC, AN EPIDEMIC, AND AN ENDEMIC?

1. Pandemic: A worldwide distribution of a disease (example: COVID-19, H1N1 influenza A virus, *Yersinia pestis* - plague)
2. Epidemic: A disease with a higher occurrence than usual, restricted to only several localities. (example: *Salmonella typhi* - Typhoid fever outbreak during 1906-1907 in the USA)
3. Endemics: A disease that is constantly present at low levels in certain localities. (example: Dengue fever is endemic in urban locations in Malaysia)

WHAT ARE THE COMMON SOURCES OF INFECTION:

1. Humans
   - Most common source of infection
2. Animals
   - Disease spread from animals are known as *zoonotic disease*
   - Example: Rabies, leptospirosis, plague
3. Insects
   - A.k.a. arthropod -borne diseases
   - Disease carrying insects are known as *vectors*

4. Soil and water
   - Soil may be contaminated with excrements of animals/birds (*Cryptococcus neoformans* – fungal/ cryptococcal meningitis)
   - Soil are also where spores of deadly bacteria are found (example: *Clostridium tetani* - tetanus, *Clostridium perfringens* - gas gangrene), they are also home to a variety of parasites (hookworms and roundworms)
   - Water can also be contaminated with bacteria (*Vibrio cholerae* - Cholera)
5. Food
   - Food poisoning (Bacteria - *Bacillus cereus, Staphylococcus aureus, Clostridium botulinum)*
   - Foodborne diseases (Bacteria - *Salmonella typhi, Escherichia coli, Shigella sp.)*

VARIOUS MODES OF DISEASE TRANSMISSION:

1. Contact
   - Can be either direct or indirect
   - Direct contact: hugging, kissing, sexual intercourse
   - Indirect contact: via inanimate objects *(fomites)* like sharing combs, toothbrush, using a pen someone with the disease has used before
2. Inhalation
   - Example: pulmonary anthrax and tuberculosis
3. Ingestion
   - Example: cholera, typhoid fever
4. Inoculation
   - To directly introduce into the body
   - Example: Rabies via bite by an infected dog, HIV by using unsterile syringes
5. Insect
   - Vector borne disease
   - Example: Dengue fever by mosquito, Lyme disease by tick bite

6. Congenital
    - a.k.a. Vertical transmission
    - Pathogens are able to cross the placental barrier from the mother to the foetus to affect it inside the uterus
    - Risks of miscarriage, stillborn or dead born increases
    - Example: congenital rubella, syphilis
7. Iatrogenic
    - Transmission occurs during medical or laboratory procedures such as lumbar puncture, injections, surgery, catheterization.

Now that we have a clear orientation of what infections are, their sources and how they transmit in general, we shall continue on to have a look at the phases of infection with respect to the general sequence of events.

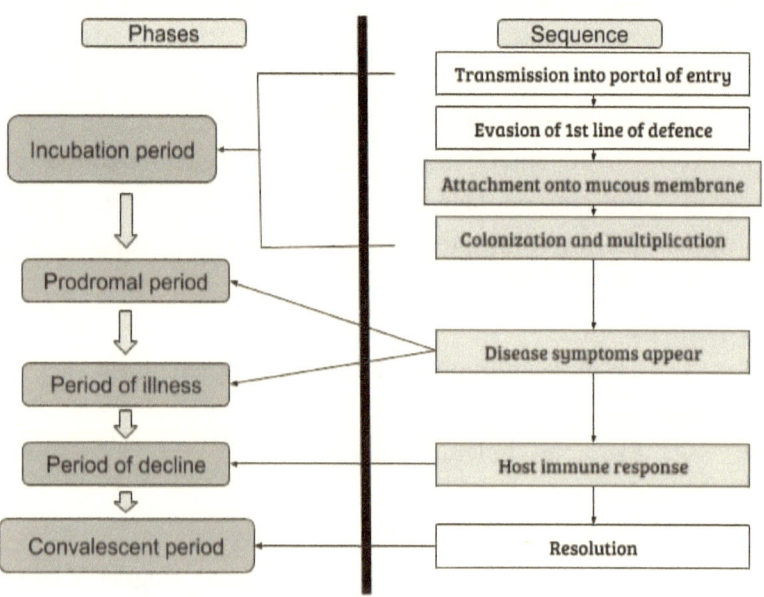

Incubation period: The duration between first exposure to a pathogen to the appearance of symptoms. Incubation period of each pathogen varies. Some may be as short as hours whereas some may take weeks to months.

Prodromal period: The time when symptoms appear but are generalized and non-specific. Meaning, it is still too early for us to determine the exact cause of the disease. Example: fever, fatigue, loss of appetite.

Period of illness: When the *pathognomonic* (specific) sign(s) and symptom(s) of the disease starts to manifest. Example: Fluid-filled, red, itchy vesicles form on the skin - chickenpox; Burning sensation upon urination with purulent (pus-like) discharge - urinary tract infection

Period of decline: The number of pathogens begin to decrease as an effective immune response is mounted. Signs and symptoms also start subsiding.

* The second and third lines of defence is mounted as soon as the first line is breached. Denoted as the highlighted boxes on the right side of the diagram.

Convalescent period: Host generally returns to normal. However, some serious diseases may cause permanent damage to certain functions of the body.

To summarize, an infection is an invasion of a pathogen into/on the body that can potentially cause a disease. In addition, there are different types of infection. We are clear with the definitions of pandemic, epidemic and endemic. We have also familiarized ourselves with the common sources and routes of transmission of infections. Lastly, the phases of infection are exposure, incubation, prodromal period, period of illness, period of decline and convalescence.

FOOD FOR THOUGHT:

We don't usually realize this until it is pointed out to us, but we humans are actually very fragile and vulnerable to everything around us. Not just immediate physical threats but to these invisible ones too. Just look at what you've come to understand so far, microorganisms are constantly seeking to exploit every vulnerability we have. The only thing that gives us a fighting chance is a remarkable defence mechanism that evolution has gifted upon mankind. Without it, we wouldn't stand a chance. The unfortunate reality is, it's very easy to destroy the only defence we have. Many a times, we do so by our own hands. You only have one, take care of it.

CHAPTER 6

Basic Bacteriology

The study of bacteria

Part 1: Characteristics of Bacteria
Part 2: Classification of Bacteria
Part 3: Bacterial Reproduction and Growth Curve
Part 4: Medically Significant Bacteria
Part 5: How Antibiotic Works

·

Summary

Part 1: Characteristics of Bacteria

When we say the word *germs*, the common visualization would be of invisible spheres and rods covering almost every surface we touch, either on our own body or on inanimate objects. We have come to know that these tiny monsters can cause serious illnesses and diseases. The things that we often picture about germs, partly thanks to commercials and advertisements of soap and body wash brands, are basically bacteria. We normally don't think further than that. This is a common misconception. Technically, the word 'germs' is a broad term that umbrellas all the different types of microorganisms. Be it bacteria, viruses, fungi etc. But here, we shall go with the general picture and talk about everyone's favourite, the bacteria.

In Chapter 1: The Basic Unit of Life, we have had an overview about the components that make up a cell. There, it was briefly mentioned that there exist two different cell types. They are the *prokaryotic cells* (a.k.a. prokaryotes) and *eukaryotic cells* (a.k.a. eukaryotes). So now, let's find out what they are.

Prokaryotes and eukaryotes are two different cell types that are differentiated by their cell structures. You can say that prokaryotes are the simpler form of cells whereas eukaryotes are much more complex. Hence, prokaryotes were the only forms of life on our planet for millennia before more complex eukaryotes came into the picture to give rise to multicellular living things like us. We can distinguish these two forms of cells by looking at their makeup. By their differences, you can easily make out how primitive prokaryotic cells are.

CHARACTERISTICS	PROKARYOTES	EUKARYOTES
Definition	*Pro* — Old *Karyone* — Nucleus Denotes the old and ancient cell type	*Eu* — New *Karyone* — Nucleus Denotes the new and more complex cell type
Cell size	0.5-3 micrometers	2-100 micrometer
Kind of cell	unicellular / single cell	Multicellular
Nucleus	• Absent • Chromosomes are condensed in a *nucleoid* — region of loosely organized DNA	• Present • Chromosomes are found in the nucleus bounded by a nuclear membrane
Nuclear membrane	Absent	Present
DNA	Circular Double stranded DNA	Linear Double stranded DNA
Number of chromosomes	Single	Multiple
Membrane bounded organelles	Absent	Present

Ribosome type	70S	80S
Mode of reproduction	Asexual	Sexual
Cell division	Binary fission	Mitosis and meiosis
Cell wall	Contains peptidoglycan	Only present in plant cells (made of cellulose) and fungi (made of chitin)
Example	Bacteria, Archaea	Plants, Animals, Fungi, Protists

By now, you should be able to tell that the cell type of what we have discussed back in Chapter 1 to be that of a eukaryote as it fulfils all the above criteria of one. Humans are made of animal cells which are in turn eukaryotes. Bacteria on the other hand are far less complicated as they were the first life on earth. Thus, they are prokaryotic cells. They fall under the domain of bacteria and the kingdom of Monera. A close look of the bacteria anatomy would reveal the following:

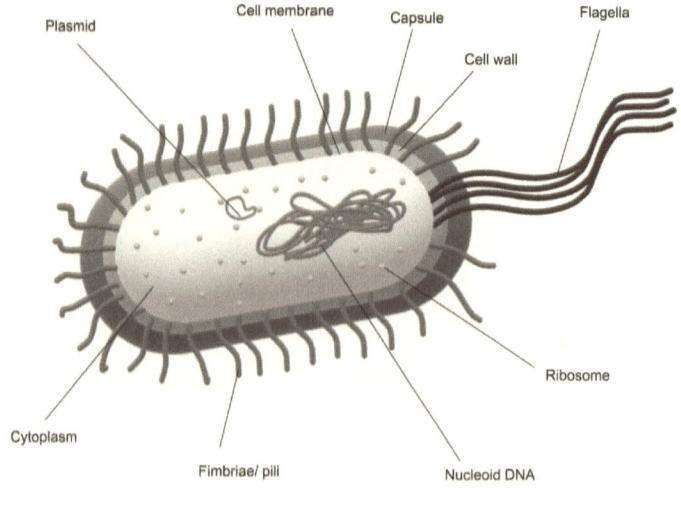

We shall now take a look into some of the structures with its function you would expect to find in bacteria other than those already mentioned in the features of a prokaryote.

STRUCTURE	DESCRIPTION AND FUNCTION
Flagellum (*plural: flagella*)	• A whip-like structure made of microtubules for locomotion • Helps in motility. • Bacteria with flagella are also called *flagellates*
Pilus (*plural: pili*) / Fimbria (*plural: fimbriae*)	• A hair-like appendage on the surface of bacteria • Helps in adhesion or attachment to another cell surface • Sex pilus acts as a conjugal bridge for genetic transfer between two bacterial cell during conjugation (a type of asexual reproduction)
Capsule	• A layer on the outer surface of the bacteria which can only be seen using specific stains • Functions to protect the cell against phagocytosis
Cell wall	• Present in prokaryotes • Made of *peptidoglycan* • It is rigid. Hence, it gives the cell support and its shape

Plasma membrane	• A phospholipid bilayer embedded with certain proteins (among them are *PBPs- Penicillin- Binding Proteins*) and enzymes
Spores	• When the environment is not conducive for the survival of the bacteria, they develop spores • Only certain bacteria are capable of forming spores. The process is known as *sporulation* • Bacterial spores are strictly meant for survival of harsh environments (unlike fungi where spores are meant for reproduction). They are highly resistant to heat, dehydration and chemicals. • They are very hard to destroy • Spores will germinate back into bacterial form when the environment becomes favourable once more.

From Chapter 4, we know that there are three domains of life and five kingdoms. Bacteria fall under the kingdom of Monera. However, within this kingdom we also find Archaea/ Archaebacteria, which belongs to an entirely different domain.

Bacteria and Archaea are both prokaryotic cells and share similar morphology but they do have some differences in properties that draw the line between the two domains of life. Simply put, the genetic makeup of Archaea varies from that of bacteria, they do not have peptidoglycan in their cell wall and they are capable of surviving in extreme environments such as in hot springs, the depths of the ocean and salt brines. In addition, archaeans are non-pathogenic. Meaning, they do not cause diseases. Because of their peculiar properties, Archaea has a completely different set of classifications than that of bacteria which we will not dive into. We are only going to focus on bacteria as they pose a potential threat to human health.

Part 2: Classification of Bacteria

We now know the importance of having everything in its place. Classification of microorganisms for the purpose of identification is of paramount importance as it could mean the difference between life and death. Imagine a highly unlikely scenario where a microbiologist could not differentiate between a gram positive coccus (spherical bacteria) from a gram positive oval budding yeast cell. Both of them look quite similar to the untrained eye. One is a bacterium and the other a fungus. He or she then reports that the ill patient is suffering from a fungal infection instead of a bacterial infection. The doctor then starts on antifungal medication. The patient did not respond to treatment and eventually succumbed to the bacterial infection. Under the microscope, the world can be a confusing place. Thankfully, scientists for generations have taken painstaking measures to identify and classify them.

Below are some of the ways bacteria are classified:

1. CLASSIFICATION ACCORDING TO *MORPHOLOGY*

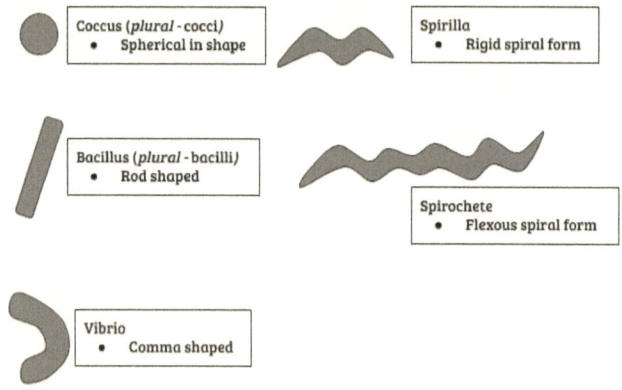

Cocci can have various arrangements. They can be in chains (Streptococci); in clusters (Staphylococci); in pairs (Diplococci) and in fours (tetrads).

Similarly, bacilli can too take up different arrangements. They can be found in chains; in clusters and in pairs (diplobacilli).

Aside from the above morphologies, there are two more:

1. Actinomycetes: They have branching filaments that look like sunrays when seen in tissue lesions
2. Mycoplasma: They are a group of bacteria that lack a cell wall and hence have no constant form or shape.

2. CLASSIFICATION ACCORDING TO *GRAM STAINING*

Gram staining is a type of staining technique developed by a Danish scientist named Hans Christian Gram. Based on the composition of the bacterial cell wall, the bacteria will either be stained *purple — gram positive* or *pink — gram negative*.

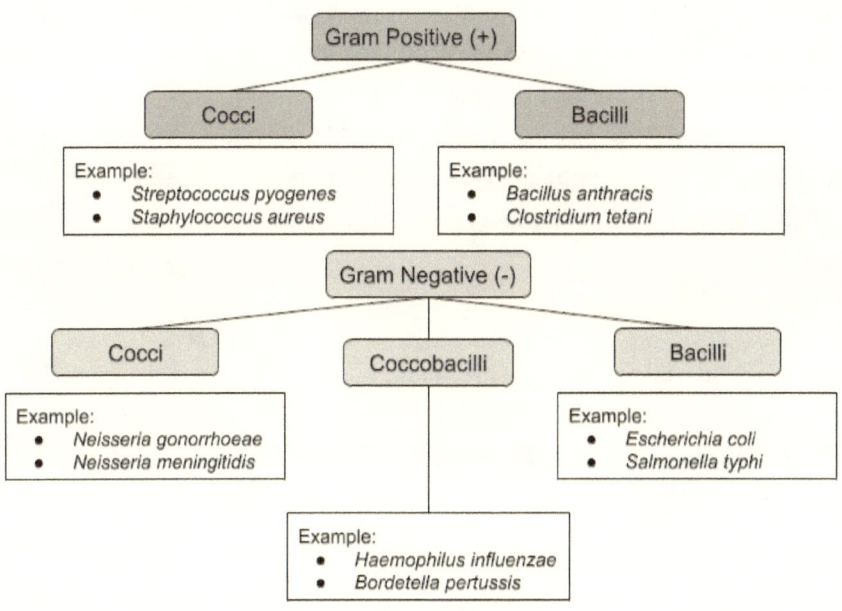

Examples:

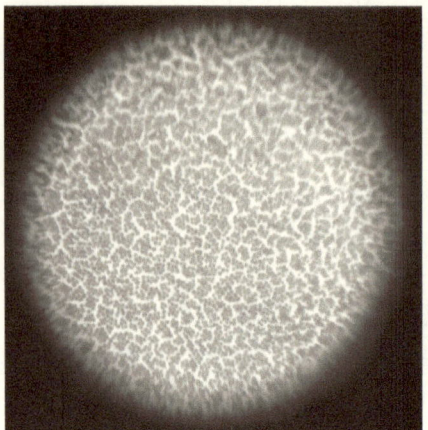 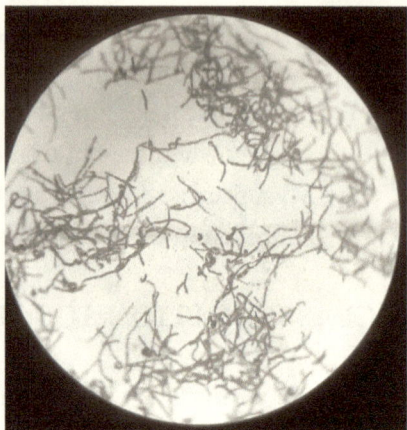

Gram positive cocci in clusters   Gram positive bacilli

It may be worth noting at this point that most gram negative (-) bacteria produces *endotoxins* that cause fever and shock (hypotension). On the other hand, *exotoxins* are produced by certain gram positive (+) and negative (-) bacteria. Its effect varies.

Not all species of bacteria can take up the gram stain. This is because they do not have the peptidoglycan component in their cell wall to take up the stain. In such cases, special stains are used.

For example:

- Acid-fast stain (Ziehl-Neelsen stain) is used to visualize *Mycobacterium tuberculosis*
- Albert stain is used to visualize *Corynebacterium diphtheriae*

3. CLASSIFICATION ACCORDING TO *OXYGEN REQUIREMENTS*

Microorganisms that require oxygen to live are called *aerobes* whereas those that do not require oxygen to live are called *anaerobes*.

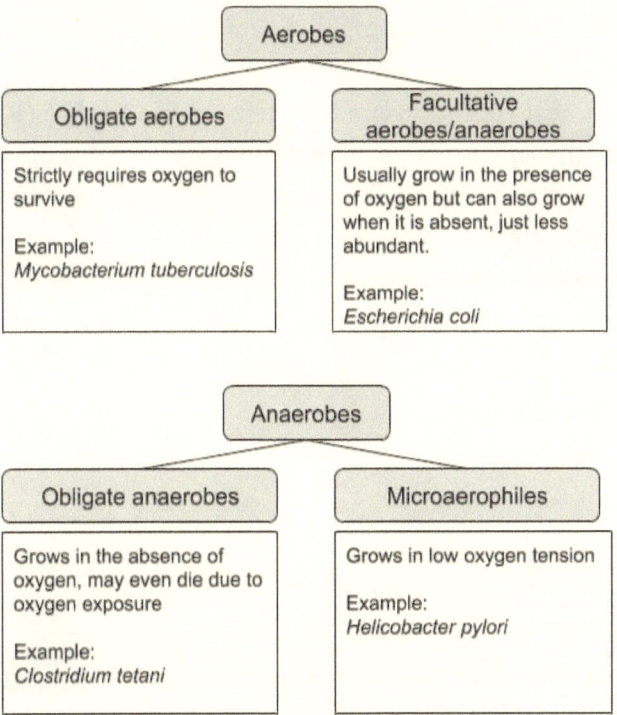

4. CLASSIFICATION ACCORDING TO *TEMPERATURE REQUIREMENTS*

Every bacterial species has their own temperature range in which they can grow. Any temperature higher or lower than their range deters growth. The specific temperature where a bacterial species thrive the most is known as the *optimum temperature.*

Most pathogenic bacteria have a temperature range that is close to the human body temperature, that is 37°C. They are called *mesophilic bacteria*. They can grow in temperatures ranging from 25°C to 40°C. An example would be *Neisseria gonorrhoeae* (30°C - 39°C).

Psychrophilic bacteria are those that can survive in temperature below 20°C, even up to -7°C. Most of which happen to be soil and water saprophytes (organisms that live on dead or decaying matter). They are generally not a concern to human health as they are mostly non-pathogenic. However, psychrophilic bacteria are responsible for food spoilage.

Bacteria that can survive in high temperatures (55°C to 80°C) are termed as *thermophiles*. A great example is *Bacillus stearothermophilus*. Again, they are mostly non-pathogenic to humans as they cannot survive in our body temperature.

Knowing the temperature range for microorganisms is important as it can help us determine the appropriate method to destroy them through sterilization.

Part 3: Bacterial Reproduction and Growth Curve

Bacteria follows an *asexual* mode of reproduction. This means that the formation of a progeny is without the fusion of two genetically different gametes. Bacteria, unlike eukaryotes, divide by *binary fission*. This means that one bacterium will split into two, then two into four, then four into eight and so on. This allows the bacteria to grow exponentially. Binary fission occurs as follows:

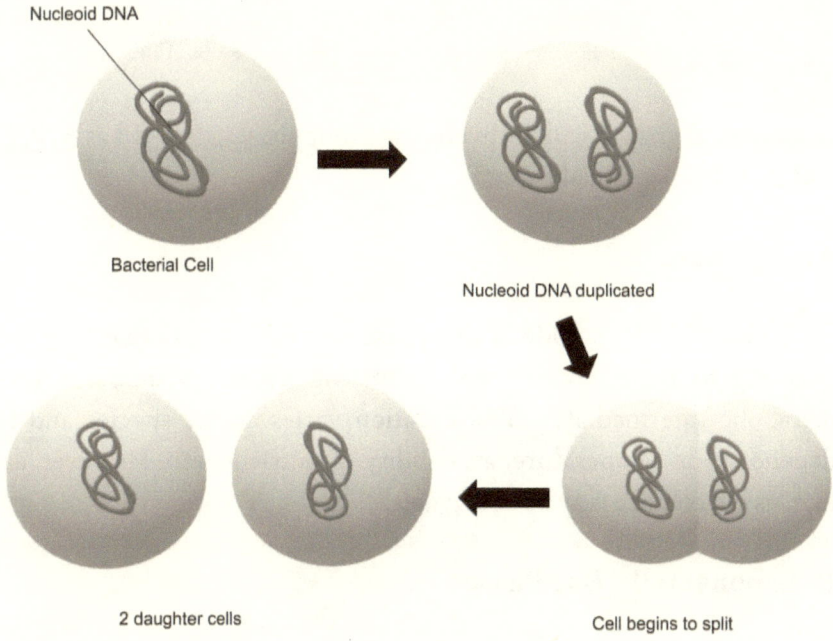

Nucleoid DNA

Bacterial Cell

Nucleoid DNA duplicated

2 daughter cells

Cell begins to split

The time it takes for one bacterial cell to become two is known as *doubling time.* Each species has their own doubling time, ranging from minutes (*E. coli*) to weeks (*M. leprae*).

If we were to culture a bacterial species on a culture media and plot the bacterial growth curve, it will look something like the graph on the next page.

BACTERIAL GROWTH CURVE

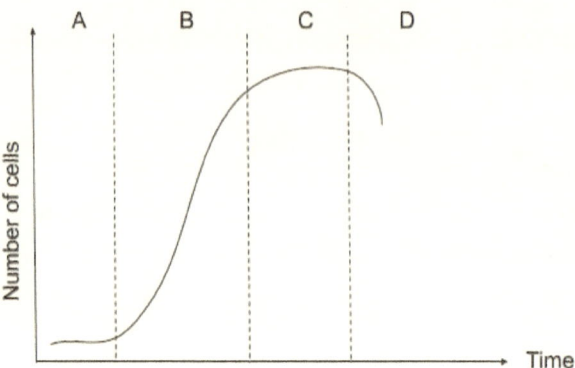

Bacterial growth can be divided into four phases, denoted as A, B, C and D in the diagram above.

A: Lag Phase

Bacteria do not divide in this phase yet. You can say that they are adapting to their environment, preparing necessary enzymes and metabolic intermediates. The duration varies across species and is dependent on temperature, availability of nutrients etc. However, an increase in cell size may be observable.

B: Exponential / Log Phase

Bacteria starts to divide rapidly and cell count increases exponentially. Cells are small and uniform in size.

C: Stationary/ Plateau Phase

After an exponential increase in number, this phase is where cell division stops due to decreased nutrients. The number of new cells are just enough to replace the number of dying cells. Sporulation (the process of forming spores) can take place in this phase.

D: Death Phase/ Phase of decline

The bacterial population starts dying due to depletion of nutrients and accumulation of toxins.

Bacteria colonies growing on culture media would look something like this:

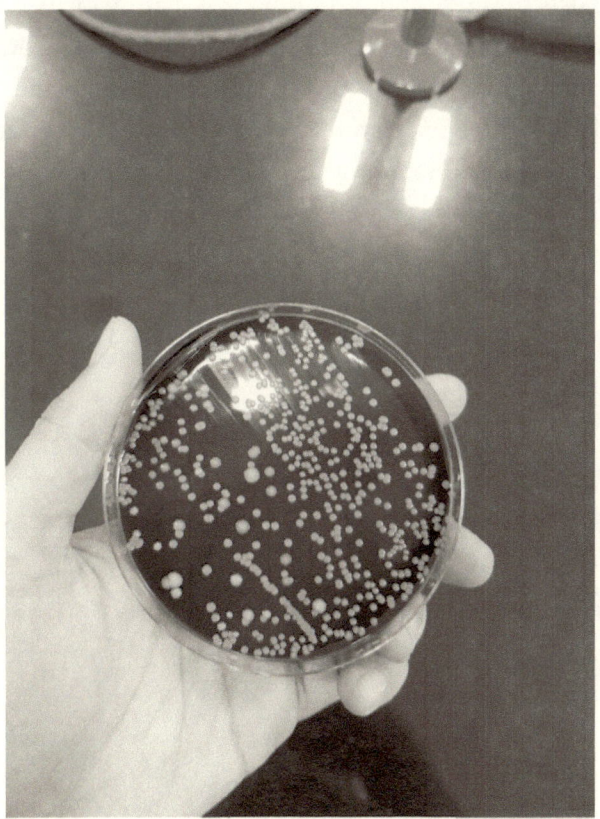

Bacteria colonies growing on a blood agar
plate (a type of culture media)

Part 4: Medically Significant Bacteria

There are multitudes of bacterial species to learn about and scientists are still uncovering new ones every day, adding on to the never-ending list. If one were to list and describe each and every different species of bacteria, it would take volumes upon volumes of textbooks to finish. Fortunately, we will not bother ourselves with bacteria that do not pose much of a significance to our human body and also not dive too much into the details of those that do. Let's leave this burden to the doctors and microbiologists to worry about. This book is mainly focussed on giving you an orientation and painting the bigger picture so that you can better understand how small things affect us. Here, you will begin to see a lot of names that may be alien to you, but it's mainly there for reference and to give you some idea. Fret not if you do not fully catch it the first time. We will first have a look at the classification of the bacteria where those which share common characteristics are clumped together. Then, we will see the diseases they cause.

The big picture for gram positive (+) bacteria:

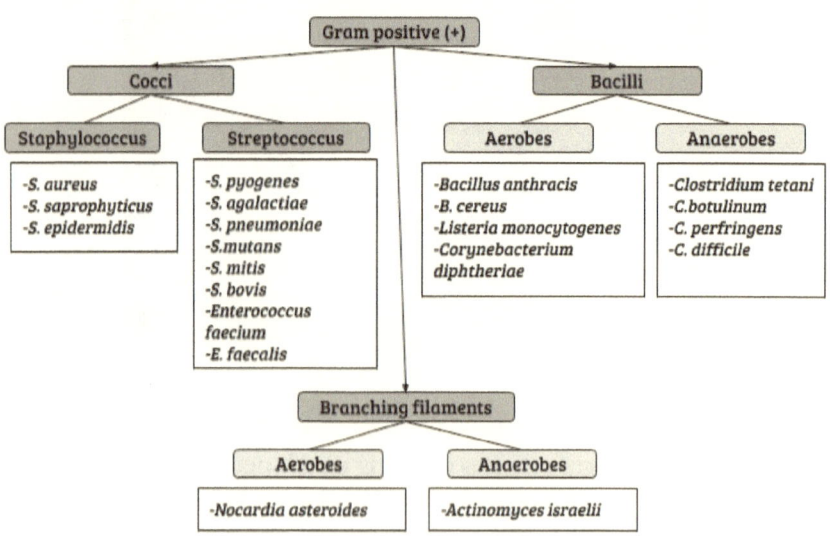

BACTERIA	DISEASE (S)
Staphylococcus aureus	• Skin diseases • Toxic shock syndrome • Food poisoning • Scalded skin syndrome
Staphylococcus saprophyticus	• Urinary tract infection (UTI)
Staphylococcus epidermidis	• Infects prosthetic implants (e.g. heart valve)
Streptococcus pyogenes	• Pharyngitis (sore throat) • Skin diseases • Toxic shock syndrome • Scarlet fever • Rheumatic heart disease • Glomerulonephritis (kidney disease)
Streptococcus agalactiae	• Meningitis in babies • Pneumonia in babies
Streptococcus mutans	• Dental caries
Streptococcus mitis	• Dental caries
Streptococcus bovis	• Subacute endocarditis (heart disease) • Colon cancer

Enterococcus faecium, E. faecalis	• UTI • Subacute endocarditis
Bacillus anthracis	• Anthrax
Bacillus cereus	• Food poisoning
Listeria monocytogenes	• Meningitis • Gastroenteritis (inflammation of gastrointestinal tract causing diarrhea-like symptoms) • Miscarriages
Corynebacterium diphtheriae	• Diphtheria
Clostridium tetani	• Tetanus
Clostridium botulinum	• Botulism
Clostridium perfringens	• Gas gangrene
Clostridium difficile	• Diarrhoea
Nocardia asteroides	• Lung infection • Skin infection
Actinomyces israelii	• Oral and facial abscess

The big picture for gram negative (-) bacteria:

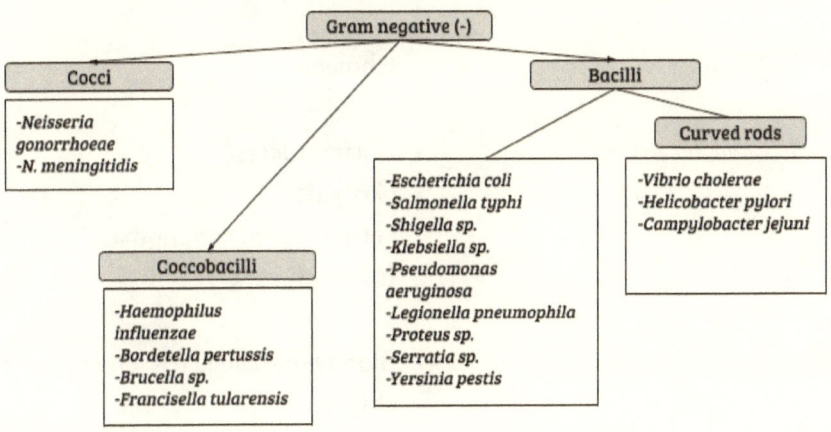

BACTERIA	DISEASE (S)
Neisseria gonorrhoeae	• Sexually transmitted disease
Neisseria meningitidis	• Meningitis • Waterhouse-Friderichsen syndrome
Haemophilus influenzae	• Pneumonia • Meningitis • Otitis media (ear infection) • Epiglottitis
Bordetella pertussis	• Pertussis/ whooping cough/ 100-day cough
Brucella sp.	• Undulating fever, night sweats, joint pain

Francisella tularensis	• Tularemia
Vibrio cholerae	• Cholera
Helicobacter pylori	• Gastric ulcers • Gastritis • Gastric adenocarcinoma (stomach cancer)
Campylobacter jejuni	• Bloody diarrhoea (dysentery) in children • Guillain-Barre syndrome • Reactive arthritis
Escherichia coli	• Diarrhoea • Dysentery • Hemolytic-uremic syndrome • UTI • Meningitis in babies
Salmonella typhi	• Typhoid fever
Shigella sp.	• Shigellosis (dysentery)
Klebsiella sp.	• Pneumonia • Abscess in lungs and liver • UTI
Legionella pneumophila	• Pneumonia

Pseadomonas aeroginosa	• Pneumonia • Sepsis • UTI • Osteomyelitis (inflammation of bone) • Otitis media • Skin infections especially on burn victims • Ecthyma gangrenosum (necrotic skin lesion)
Proteus sp.	• UTI
Serratia sp.	• Pneumonia • UTI
Yersinia pestis	• Plague

Bacteria not observable by gram staining include:

1. MYCOBACTERIA

BACTERIA	DISEASE (S)
Mycobacterium tuberculosis	• Tuberculosis
Mycobacterium leprae	• Leprosy

2. MYCOPLASMA

BACTERIA	DISEASE (S)
Mycoplasma pneumoniae	• Pneumonia

3. SPIROCHETES

BACTERIA	DISEASE (S)
Treponema pallidum	• Syphilis
Borrelia burgdorferi	• Lyme disease
Borrelia recurrentis	• Relapsing fever
Leptospira interrogans	• Leptospirosis

4. CHLAMYDIAE

BACTERIA	DISEASE (S)
C. trachomatis	• Urethritis • Pneumonia • Conjunctivitis • Trachoma • Lymphogranuloma venereum
C. pneumoniae	• Pneumonia
C. psittaci	• Psittacosis (pneumonia)

5. RICKETTSIAE

BACTERIA	DISEASE (S)
R. rickettsii, R. akari	• Spotted fever

R. prowazekii, R. typhi, R. tsutsugamushi	• Typhus group of diseases
Coxiella burnetii	• Q fever

Don't be alarmed if you cannot remember everything mentioned for the past few pages. Even medical students take a whole year to master it.

Before we bring this part of the chapter to an end, there is one more subject that has to be brought to attention. And that is the existence of something called *serotypes*.

Serotypes or serovars are groups within a bacterial or viral species that possess distinctive surface structures. Remember how different organisms can be differentiated into various categories based on shared characteristics? This forms the entire basis of taxonomy. For example, if we look at Haemophilus influenzae under the microscope, you will find that the cells look indistinguishable from one another. They are all gram negative coccobacilli. However, they actually differ in surface antigens (proteins) that necessitates a subspecies level of differentiation. We call this, serotyping. Consider the following analogy:

Imagine you are an advanced alien civilization visiting planet Earth for the first time. From space, you peer through your telescope and discover the existence of the human species, *Homo sapiens*. From afar, you noticed humans all look similar, a head with four limbs connected to a trunk, walking upright, minding their own business. You decided you wanted to come down to Earth to visit the place. On your journey across the globe, you realized that not all humans are the same. Their skin tone differs from continent to continent. You later learnt that the human species have different races.

Similarly, a single bacterial species can have multiple serotypes depending on the type and number of surface antigens on said bacterial cell.

For instance:

Haemophilus influenzae has six different serotypes: a - f where b causes the most severe disease.

Neisseria meningitidis has thirteen known serotypes where group A, B, C, Y and W are the most common cause of disease.

Serotypes are of great significance when it comes to developing vaccines. Smallpox happened to be the only human disease successfully eradicated from the face of the Earth mainly owing to the fact that the virus that caused it only had one serotype. Therefore, a vaccine against one serotype of the smallpox virus can grant complete immunity against the disease. In contrast - continuing with the example of *H. influenzae*, there is only a vaccine against *H. influenzae* type B (HiB) which offers us protection against it. But this vaccine is ineffective against other serotypes, a, c, d, e and f.

Part 5: How Antibiotics Work

The 28th of September 1928 was a day that revolutionized the entire medical field. A wonder drug was discovered. By accident! Alexander Fleming was a Scottish physician/scientist born in 1881. While researching staphylococci, he left a petri dish of it uncovered near an open window. The plate got contaminated with a species of fungi later known to be under the genus *Penicillium,* a mold. Fleming noticed that the gram positive bacteria surrounding the contaminant died. It was then discovered that the mold secreted some kind of substance that killed the bacteria. This substance turned out to be man's first ever antibiotic, later known as *penicillin.* Since its discovery, penicillin has saved millions of lives every year and opened a new path in the field of medicine leading to the development of more antibiotics. Many people used to die after getting serious bacterial infections but with these bacteria killers, the human race suddenly stand a fighting chance.

Nowadays, doctors prescribe various types of antibiotics when a bacterial infection is diagnosed. Knowing the mechanism of how each class of antibiotics work helps in its selection to treat the disease.

The bookish definition of an antibiotic is defined as a substance produced by a microorganism that is capable of inhibiting and killing other microorganisms. They can be classified based on their spectrum of action or whether they inhibit or kill the microorganism.

Broad-spectrum antibiotics kill a wide range of bacteria which include gram negative bacteria, gram positive bacteria and others like rickettsia and chlamydia.

On the other hand, *narrow-spectrum antibiotics* are effective against a limited number of bacteria.

If an antibiotic works by *killing off* the bacteria, they are known to be *bactericidal* whereas those that work by *inhibiting its continual growth* are said to be *bacteriostatic* antibiotics.

As mentioned, different classes of antibiotics have a different mechanism and site of action. The following diagram will illustrate the different antibiotics with its site of action.

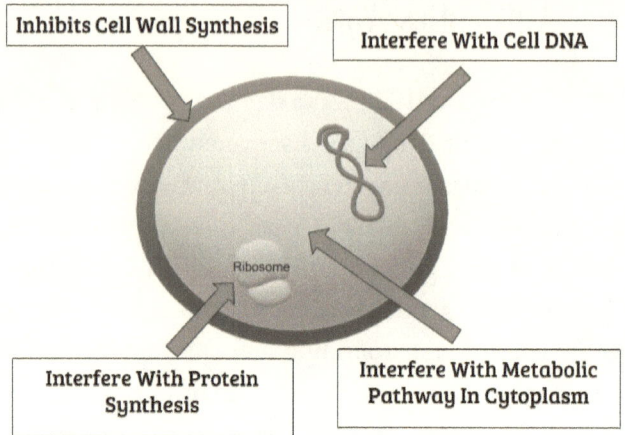

MECHANISM OF ACTION OF VARIOUS ANTIBIOTIC CLASSES WITH EXAMPLES:

1. Inhibits cell wall synthesis

CLASS	EXAMPLES
β(beta) - lactams	Penicillin, Amoxicillin, Ceftriaxone, Imipenems, Aztrionam
Glycopeptides	Vancomycin, Teicoplanin
Bacitracin	-

2. Interferes with protein synthesis in the ribosome

CLASS	EXAMPLES
Aminoglycosides	Gentamicin, Streptomycin, Neomycin

Tetracyclines	Tetracycline, Doxycycline, Minocycline
Macrolides	Azithromycin, Erythromycin, Clarithromycin
Chloramphenicol	-
Lincosamides	Lincomycin, Clindamycin
Oxazolidinones	Linezolid, Radezolid

3. Interferes with the various metabolic pathways of the bacterial cell

CLASS	EXAMPLES
Sulfonamides	Sulfamethoxazole, Sulfadoxine, Sulfadiazine
Trimethoprim	-

4. Interferes at the DNA level

CLASS	EXAMPLES
Fluoroquinolones	Ciprofloxacin, Norfloxacin, Levofloxacin
Rifampin	A.k.a. Rifampicin

Due to the overuse of antibiotics, many strains of antibiotic-resistant bacteria have emerged. Bacteria that are not completely killed off during the course of an antibiotic therapy will 'learn' and mutate into strains that are resistant. Thus, the use of stronger antibiotics is necessary as the previous one is no longer effective in killing them. Bacteria that are resistant to more than one class of antibiotics are known as *Multi-Drug Resistant* (MDR) bacteria. Recently, even *Extensively- Drug Resistant* (XDR) bacteria have also emerged as seen in *Mycobacterium tuberculosis* (causes TB). These 'superbugs' pack a huge punch to the face as doctors struggle to cure their patients due to the limited choices of drugs they can use. Our miracle drug is failing us and if we don't do something to overcome this problem, we risk falling back to an age before the discovery of penicillin.

The general public's actions to help curb the emergence of drug resistant bacteria are tantamount to pharmaceutical efforts in developing stronger drugs. As such, people should:

1. finish the prescribed course of antibiotic treatment.
2. not buy antibiotics for self-treatment as they are prescription drugs.
3. not demand for antibiotics from your physician if he/she deems it unnecessary. Antibiotics, as you now know, are only effective against a bacterial infection. No benefit will come out of taking it in case of diseases caused by viral infection.
4. spread awareness of this knowledge to family and friends and see to it that they participate in the fight against drug resistant microorganisms.

Basic Bacteriology Summary

- Bacteria are prokaryotic cells belonging to the Bacteria domain and Monera kingdom.
- The bacteria anatomy share several special features: flagella, pili, capsule, cell wall, spores etc.
- Bacteria can be classified based on their morphology, gram staining, oxygen requirements and temperature requirements.
- Bacteria reproduce asexually through binary fission. This allows an exponential growth. When plotted on a graph, their growth curve can be divided into four phases: lag phase, log/exponential phase, stationary/ plateau phase and lastly, phase of decline.
- Bacteria that can cause human diseases are of medical importance and a good number of them have been listed in Part 4.
- Antibiotics are substances produced by a microorganism that kills other microorganisms. They are classified as either broad or narrow spectrum antibiotics; as bactericidal or bacteriostatic antibiotics. Different classes of antibiotics work through different mechanisms. They interfere with cell wall synthesis; interfere with protein synthesis; interfere with metabolic pathways; or interfere at the level of DNA. Antibiotics only work against bacteria and are ineffective against viruses, fungi, protozoa, and parasites.

FOOD FOR THOUGHT:

It's intriguing to think that Archaea and Bacteria were the first forms of life from which all complex multicellular organisms alive today stem from. If we trace back the branches of the metaphorical tree of life down to its roots, you will find these primitive cells. Isn't it a wonderful thing to be part of this beautiful picture. From nothingness, dust and dirt, whether by accident or design, generated simple mechanics to support life. And we, humans, are the same dust in the highest exalted form. It is important for us as a species to look forward and move on but it is also equally important to reminisce our humble beginnings and be thankful for what we have become. The tree of life shows us that all life is connected and we are all made of the same thing. This might be speaking the obvious but the sad truth is, not everybody realizes it as we are too caught up with the rapidly changing world. We have a shared responsibility to care not just for ourselves, but also for every life there is on this planet. If you admit humans are the epitome of evolution, then with great power comes great responsibilities.

CHAPTER 7

Basic Mycology

The study of fungi

Part 1: Characteristics of Fungi
Part 2: Classification of Fungi
Part 3: Medically Significant Fungi
Part 4: How Antifungal Drugs Work

.

Summary

Part 1: Characteristics of Fungi

If you could recall the short story of John in the introduction of the book, you would remember that the bread he was about to eat for breakfast did not successfully make the journey down his gut. Instead, it went straight to the bin. John saw mold growing on it and decided he didn't want to risk having an upset stomach. We're all too familiar with this scenario. How many times have we noticed black-green patches growing on our baked goods? Sometimes, we see them even on rotting fruits and vegetables. Generally, people call them mold. But molds are actually a class of fungi.

Aren't fungi big observable structures (macroscopic) like mushrooms? That's not entirely wrong. This just isn't the big picture. Among the five kingdoms of life, fungi are one of them. It's normally used as an umbrella term that covers all types of mushrooms, molds and yeasts. Based on this, we now know the existence of macroscopic multicellular fungi (e.g. mushrooms) and microscopic unicellular fungi (e.g. yeast). Classification of fungi will be discussed in Part 2 of this chapter. As of now, we must be well familiarized with the common characteristics shared among fungi.

Common traits of fungi include:

- They are all eukaryotic cells.
- They can present as unicellular or multicellular organisms.
- Their cell wall is made of *chitin* (a long chain polymer made of polysaccharides, derived from glucose).
- Their cell membrane contains *ergosterol.*
- They lack chlorophyll. In other words, fungi do not synthesize their own food. Fungi are known as *heterotrophs* (*hetero* - others). Heterotrophs are organisms that cannot make their own food and derive nutrients from other organisms. Examples of other heterotrophs are humans and animals.
- They are capable of producing spores as means of reproduction. Fungi can reproduce sexually as well as asexually.
- Some species are thermally dimorphic. Meaning, they are capable of changing forms/shapes in different temperature settings.

A good majority of fungi are obligate aerobes whereas some are facultative aerobes. One thing is certain, no fungal species are ever obligate anaerobic. Because fungi are heterotrophs and require a source of carbon, they are ubiquitous in the environment, especially among the dead and decaying matter. Fungi are responsible for food spoilage but at the same time can be used in the preparation of food. For example, yeasts are used in the process of baking bread and brewing wine.

Some features of fungi are opposites of those found in bacteria. It's not uncommon to compare the two because of its contrasting characteristics. Since our last chapter was on bacteria, the following table summarizes the differences seen between the two kingdoms for revision.

CHARACTERISTICS	FUNGI	BACTERIA
Size	~ 4 micrometers	~ 1 micrometer
Cell type	Eukaryote	Prokaryote
Organelles	Membrane bounded organelles present	Membrane bounded organelles absent
Cell membrane	Contains *ergosterol*	Contains cholesterol - except *Mycoplasma*
Cell wall	Made of chitin	Made of peptidoglycan
Spore formation	For reproduction	For survival
Mode of reproduction	Sexual and asexual	Asexual
Thermally dimorphic	Yes (certain species)	No

People often get confused between algae and fungi. Many associate them to be the same but in reality, they are not. Although they do share certain characteristics, they belong to different kingdoms altogether. Algae, by definition, are eukaryotic organisms (except blue-green algae a.k.a. Cyanobacteria which are prokaryotes) belonging to the kingdom Protista that are capable of photosynthesis but lack the reproductive structures of plants.

Unlike fungi, algae are *autotrophs* because they make their own food as they contain chloroplast for photosynthesis. The major reason algae do not come under the kingdom Plantae is because they do not possess plant structures like roots, stems and leaves. Like plants, algae contribute in releasing oxygen into Earth's atmosphere. As a matter of fact, algae are believed to be the organism responsible for turning a once inhabitable Earth into a planet where complex life was able to thrive. Around six hundred fifty million years ago, life on infant Earth was restricted to simple organisms like bacteria floating around in the sea. It was due to an algae bloom that produced an abundance of oxygen in Earth's atmosphere that created the stepping stone for the formation of a higher and complex life forms. Besides, algae are the primary producers in the aquatic food chain.

For comparison, the table below summarizes the differences between fungi and algae. This should be sufficient to clear doubts and confusion in distinguishing the two.

CHARACTERISTICS	ALGAE	FUNGI
Kingdom	Protista	Fungi
Habitat	Aquatic— fresh and marine water	Terrestrial—on decaying matter

Cell type	Eukaryotic (mostly; except cyanobacteria—prokaryotic)	Eukaryotic
Presence of chlorophyll	• Present • Can synthesize own food • Autotrophic • Can only survive in the presence of light	• Absent • Cannot synthesize own food • Heterotrophic • Can survive without the presence of light

Part 2: Classification of Fungi

The kingdom Fungi can be further subdivided into five phyla based on their mode of reproduction. They are:

1. Chytridiomycota
2. Zygomycota
3. Ascomycota
4. Basidiomycota
5. Glomeromycota
6. Deuteromycota (an informal group of unrelated fungi that reproduces asexually.)

Fungi reproduce sexually. They do so by mating and forming sexual spores. Its process of sexual reproduction is unique for every phyla and hence we shall not concern ourselves too much with the details. Fungi under the phylum Deuteromycota do not propagate sexually. Hence, they are otherwise known as 'imperfect fungi'. A good number of fungal species that are of medical relevance reproduce asexually by forming *conidia* (asexual spores).

One way of asexual reproduction undertaken by fungi, other than forming asexual spores is through the process of *budding* as shown below:

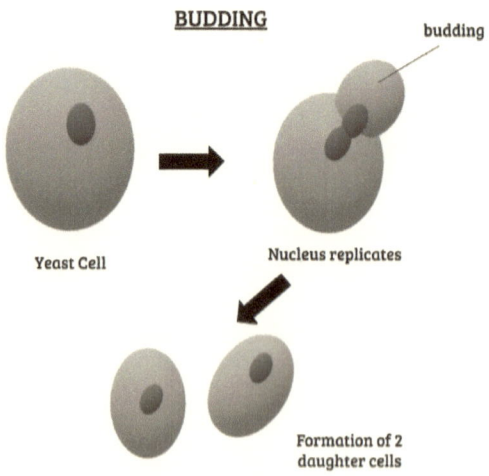

BUDDING

budding

Yeast Cell

Nucleus replicates

Formation of 2 daughter cells

Not all fungi are pathogenic to human beings. Those that are of medical significance can be easily classified in two ways:

1. **CLASSIFICATION ACCORDING TO *MORPHOLOGY*:**

MORPHOLOGY	DESCRIPTION	EXAMPLE
Yeast	• Unicellular • Stained as gram positive (+) oval budding yeast cells • Reproduces asexually by budding.	• *Cryptococcus neoformans*
Yeast-like	• Unicellular • Stained as gram positive (+) oval budding yeast cells • Reproduces asexually by budding. • Can form pseudohyphae	• *Candida albicans*
Mold	• Multicellular • Grows as long filaments called hyphae and forms a mat known as mycelium • Hyphae may be septate (have transverse walls) or aseptate (does not have transverse walls)	• *Mucor spp.*

Dimorphic	• Multicellular • Present as mold form in the environment (~25°C) but in yeast form in body tissue or at 37°C	• *Histoplasma capsulatum*

2. CLASSIFICATION ACCORDING TO TYPES OF INFECTION

Fungal infections are medically known as mycoses. The diagram below shows the different types of mycoses with examples.

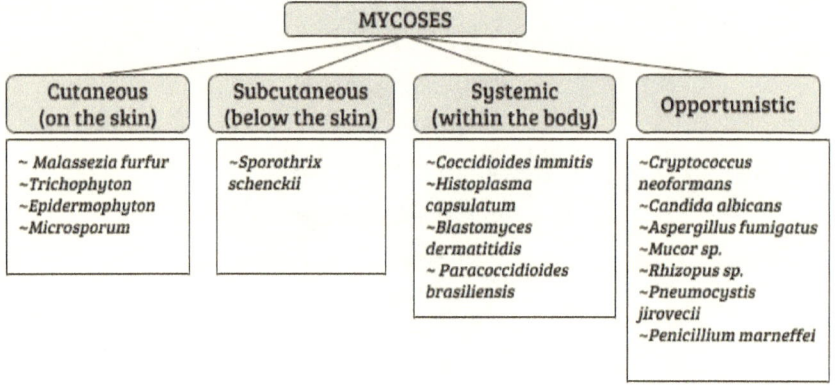

MYCOSES			
Cutaneous (on the skin)	**Subcutaneous (below the skin)**	**Systemic (within the body)**	**Opportunistic**
~ *Malassezia furfur* ~*Trichophyton* ~*Epidermophyton* ~*Microsporum*	~*Sporothrix schenckii*	~*Coccidioides immitis* ~*Histoplasma capsulatum* ~*Blastomyces dermatitidis* ~ *Paracoccidioides brasiliensis*	~*Cryptococcus neoformans* ~*Candida albicans* ~*Aspergillus fumigatus* ~*Mucor sp.* ~*Rhizopus sp.* ~*Pneumocystis jirovecii* ~*Penicillium marneffei*

Part 3: Medically Significant Fungi

When we, especially the lay people think of an infection in the body, fungi would probably not even make the list of likely causes. The manifestation of a fungal infection is not always obvious to the untrained eye unless you know what you're looking for. A few examples of a fungal infection some of us may have experienced are:

1. Ringworms — this is a fungal infection of the skin caused by dermatophytes. The term 'ringworm' is a misnomer as it is in fact, not caused by worms although its manifestation on the skin may look like it.
2. Tinea unguium — otherwise known as *onychomycosis*. This is a fungal infection of the nail(s). Characterized by a yellowish-brown discolouration, thickening of the nail and at times, separation of nail from the nail bed. It mostly affects toenails.

Therefore, this chapter aims to give you a brief idea of mycoses caused by certain fungal species of medical relevance with regards to the type of infection, anatomical location affected and key clinical presentations of the disease.

CUTANEOUS (ON THE SKIN) INFECTIONS:

CAUSATIVE AGENT	ANATOMICAL LOCATION	DISEASE	CLINICAL PRESENTATION
Malassezia furfur	Keratin layer of the skin (dead layer)	Tinea versicolor	• White discolouration of the skin (hypopigmentation)

Microsporum, Trichophyton, Epidermophyton (these are genus of the causative agent)	• Hair • Skin • Nails	Dermatophytosis (ringworms)	• Ring of inflammatory and pruritic(itchy) vesicles

SUBCUTANEOUS (UNDERNEATH THE SKIN) INFECTIONS:

CAUSATIVE AGENT	ANATOMICAL LOCATION	DISEASE	CLINICAL PRESENTATION
Sporothrix schenckii	Subcutaneous tissue	Sporotrichosis	• Local pustules or ulcers • Nodules along draining lymphatics • Painless • Often seen in gardeners where thorn prick introduces the mold under the skin.

SYSTEMIC INFECTIONS: affects the organ(s) of the body.

CAUSATIVE AGENT	DISEASE	CLINICAL PRESENTATION
Coccidioides immitis	Coccidioidomycosis	• Valley fever • Fungus disseminates to bone and meninges in those who are pregnant and whose immunity is compromised

Histoplasma capsulatum	Histoplasmosis	• Cavities in the lungs • Granulomas in liver and spleen • Decreased RBC, WBC, platelet count • Tongue ulcers in those with compromised immunity
Blastomyces dermatitidis	Blastomycosis	• Ulcers on skin
Paracoccidioides brasiliensis	Paracoccidioidomycosis	• Ulcers on face and mouth

OPPORTUNISTIC INFECTIONS:

CAUSATIVE AGENT	ANATOMICAL LOCATION	DISEASE	CLINICAL PRESENTATION
Cryptococcus neoformans	Meninges	Cryptococcosis	• Meningitis: fever, headache, neck stiffness
Candida albicans	Multi-organ involvement: mouth, oesophagus, heart, skin, vagina etc.	Candidiasis	• Oral and/or vaginal thrush • Endocarditis (heart) • Onychomycosis • Diaper rash
Aspergillus fumigatus	• Skin • Eyes • Ears • Lungs	Aspergillosis	• Fungus ball in lungs • Sinusitis • Wound infection

Mucor sp. & Rhizopus sp.	• Paranasal air sinuses • Lungs • Gut	Mucormycosis	• Necrosis and infarction of tissues (death of tissue) due to blocked blood vessels
Pneumocystis jirovecii	• Lungs		• Fever • Pneumonia • Cough • Difficult breathing • Mortality is high in patients with AIDS

Part 4: How Antifungal Drugs Work?

Just like how most drugs work, antifungal agents are designed to kill or inhibit fungal growth by exploiting the knowledge of the structures and chemical processes of fungi. If a single component of the structure, take ergosterol for example, is disrupted, then the integrity of the cell membrane would be compromised. Eventually, this leads to the cells' death. Likewise, there are several other components and chemical pathways in the fungi that can be disrupted to contribute to therapeutic success.

The diagram below portrays the mechanism of action of several antifungal medications.

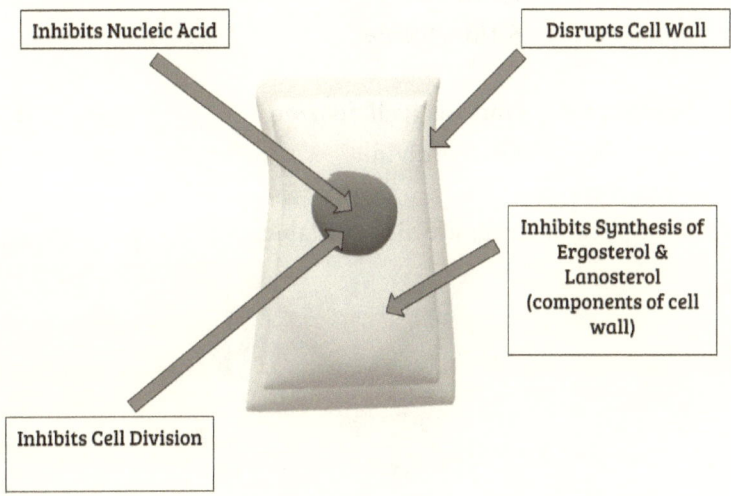

Inhibits Nucleic Acid

Disrupts Cell Wall

Inhibits Synthesis of Ergosterol & Lanosterol (components of cell wall)

Inhibits Cell Division

MECHANISM OF ACTION OF ANTIFUNGAL DRUGS WITH EXAMPLES:

1. Binds to ergosterol in the fungal cell membrane and increase membrane permeability by forming pores, causing leakage of cellular ions and other molecules.

   Example: Amphotericin B

   Nystatin

2. Inhibits the synthesis of ergosterol.
    Example: Clotrimazole
                    Ketoconazole
                    Fluconazole
                    Itraconazole

3. Inhibits the synthesis of lanosterol and ergosterol.
    Example: Terbinafine

4. Inhibits synthesis of fungal cell wall.
    Example: Caspofungin
                    Micafungin

5. Inhibits DNA synthesis.
    Example: 5-flucytosine

6. Inhibits fungal mitosis (cell division).
    Example: Griseofulvin

*Topically applicable drugs are also available.

Basic Mycology Summary

- Fungi are eukaryotic cells belonging to the Eukarya domain under the kingdom Fungi.
- Fungi can be unicellular or multicellular. Unlike bacteria, they have chitin in their cell wall, ergosterol in their plasma membrane, and forms spores as means of reproduction. Fungi can reproduce sexually as well as asexually.
- Fungi can be classified based on their morphology (yeast, yeast-like, mold and dimorphic fungi) and types of infection caused (cutaneous, subcutaneous, systemic and opportunistic).
- Fungi that can cause human diseases are of medical importance and a good number of them have been listed in Part 3.
- Antifungal medications work by inhibiting certain structures and chemical processes that are essential for the survival and growth of the fungi.

FOOD FOR THOUGHT:

Visuals of fungi may appear gruesome and disturbing to some. Many even associate them with thoughts of rotting and decaying matter. However, the contributions of fungi to humans and other life on earth are just as plentiful. From the first baked leavened bread to when grapes first transformed into wine, we humans have been indirectly aware of the actions of fungi around us. In fact, they can be found almost everywhere, just like bacteria, lurking in the air, soil, water bodies, food and even inside us. Other than being used in fermentation of food, farming and as a potential biological insecticide, fungi are equally important to the medical field. One of the most famous examples was the discovery of penicillin, a bacterium killing agent produced from a fungus. A reflection that can be made here is that good can be found even in the worst of circumstances. There are always pros and cons to things in life and it is up to ourselves to decide what we plan to focus on and make of the situation. Fungi may be thought of as the bad guy which destroys and eats away but without them, many things won't be possible, even our existence. It often takes little and small things to show us, big people, that life is how we choose to see it.

CHAPTER 8

Basic Virology

The study of viruses

Part 1: Characteristics of Viruses
Part 2: Replication of Viruses
Part 3: Classification of Viruses
Part 4: Medically Significant Viruses
Part 5: How Antiviral Drugs work

·

Summary

Part 1: Characteristics of Viruses

The word 'virus' has been all the rage these days. Amidst the COVID-19 pandemic that brought many countries to their knees when 2020 was encroaching its midpoint, the word virus portrayed various meanings to different people. Some see it as a threat to human health and couldn't be more cautious about personal hygiene. Others find it overrated, thinking that the world is giving too much publicity than it deserves to the extent that they become complacent about safety measures and put others in jeopardy. Whatever your views about the virus may be, this current pandemic (at the time of writing) has no doubt brought upon an immeasurable negative impact socially, economically and psychologically on a global scale.

Compared to other microorganisms that we have come to learn so far, none has the capability to spread as rapidly as a virus and result in that much damage. Unlike bacteria, fungi and parasites, viruses are practically useless on their own. This is because a virus is not a cell and neither is it made of cells. And we know by now that cells are the most basic unit of life as it is capable of carrying out essential processes to support life. As a matter of fact, there's this huge controversy to even call a virus a living organism. Multiple literatures place viruses in the grey area where life and death overlaps. This is because a virus requires a host cell to replicate, making more copies of itself to spread and infect even more cells. Most of the time at the end of the process, the host cell dies. You can think of them as tiny chemical components that invade and take advantage of a host's biological machinery to create progenies. Much like how a computer virus is a programme that condemns your computer. Hence, Marc H. V. van Regenmortel, a virologist from the University of Strasbourg in France and Brian W. J. Mahy of the CDC (Centers for Disease Control and Prevention) have poetically described viruses as *a kind of borrowed life* based on their dependence on a host cell.

Viruses are submicroscopic. This means that if you were to view them under a conventional microscope, you would find absolutely nothing. Bacteria are considered giants to the virus. The average size of a bacterium is around one thousand nanometers in length whereas the virus only ranges from twenty to two hundred fifty nanometers. To put things into perspective, if a fully grown adult human being is a bacterium, then a virus would be the size of a mouse. Only with the aid of an electron microscope can scientists visualize what viruses look like. Some are spherical; some spiky; some look like a crown while some resemble a worm. All in all, they are terrifyingly captivating.

There are different families of viruses, each with their own unique features. That will be discussed in Part 3 of this chapter. However, the common characteristics shared by all viruses are as follows:

- They do not possess a cellular organization. It is established that viruses are not cells so they lack all the organelles.
- They either contain DNA (deoxyribonucleic acid) or RNA (ribonucleic acid) as their genetic material, but *never* both as seen in other cellular organisms be it bacteria, fungi or parasites.
- It is obligatory for them to infect a host cell in order to replicate and spread. In order words, they are useless, lifeless and have no metabolic activity outside a host.
- They multiply through a rather complex process and not by binary fission or budding.
- They are resistant to antibiotics. This is medically significant.
- Unlike bacteria or fungi where scientists can grow them on an inanimate (non-living) culture media, viruses cannot be grown by the same method. They are grown in a cell culture. For example, they can be grown in eggs.

A virus typically has four important structures:

STRUCTURE	DESCRIPTION & FUNCTION
Core	• Contains the viral nucleic acid (genetic material) • Either a DNA or an RNA
Capsid	• It is a protein coat that surrounds the core • It forms an impenetrable shell around the core • They can take up various shapes such as *icosahedral* (cubical), *helical* and *complex* • The viral core and the capsid are collectively known as the *nucleocapsid* • It functions to protect the nucleic acid from inactivation by deleterious agents in the environment • It also adheres to host cell surfaces and introduces the viral nucleic acid into the cell
Envelope	• Depending on the family the virus hails from, it may or may not possess an envelope • It is derived from the host cell membrane and made of lipoprotein • Lipid is of the host origin but the proteins are encoded by the virus • They confer chemical, antigenic and biologic properties on the viruses
Viral proteins	• Forms structures (e.g. capsid) and enzymes that help regulate the processes of infection and replication

The diagram below shows a virus from the Herpes Family for the purpose of illustrating the important viral structures discussed earlier.

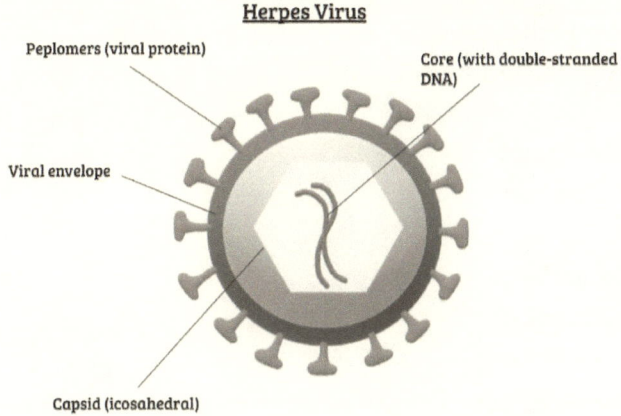

Herpes Virus

Peplomers (viral protein)

Core (with double-stranded DNA)

Viral envelope

Capsid (icosahedral)

To give you a better picture of how viruses differ from other cellular organisms, a bacterium for example, the table below shows the comparison between the two.

PROPERTY	VIRUS	BACTERIA
Nucleic acid	DNA or RNA	Both DNA and RNA
Membrane	Some may have lipoprotein envelope	Has a phospholipid bilayer as cell membrane
Ribosome	Absent	Present
Enzyme	Few if not none	Present and many
Replication	Lytic or lysogenic cycle	Binary fission

Part 2: Replication of Viruses

As mentioned in Part 1, a virus is an obligate intracellular agent that requires a host cell to produce progenies. There are six basic stages to viral replication and they are as follows:

1. Attachment
2. Penetration
3. Uncoating
4. Biosynthesis
5. Maturation
6. Release

We shall look into each stage of viral replication in a little more detail with pictorial aids.

ATTACHMENT

- The virus comes into contact with a cell by random collision.
- The virus binds to specific receptor sites on the host's cell membrane.
- This interaction between the virus and the receptors found on the host cell is highly specific as it determines the type of cells the virus can infect.
- For example, Hepatitis viruses can only infect liver cells (a.k.a hepatocytes) and not other cells.
- This is analogous to how specific keys are needed to open specific locks.

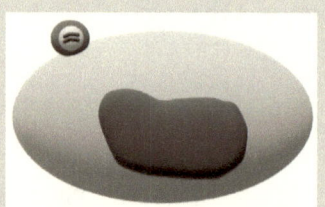

Replication of an enveloped virus:

PENETRATION

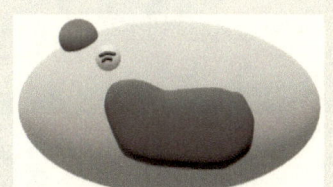

- It is the process whereby the viral genetic material is introduced into the host cell.
- Viral particles may be engulfed by the cell through a mechanism resembling phagocytosis, known as *viropexis*.
- In an enveloped virus, the lipoprotein envelope fuses with the cell membrane of the host cell and the viral nucleocapsid is released into the host cell's cytoplasm.

UNCOATING

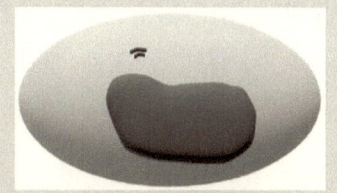

- This is the process where the virus is stripped off its outer layers (including the capsid) to expose the nucleic acid core.

BIOSYNTHESIS

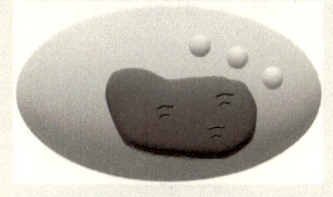

- The viral nucleic acid 'hijacks' the cell's biological machinery to code and synthesize parts (nucleic acid, capsid protein, enzymes etc.) needed to create more copies of itself.

MATURATION

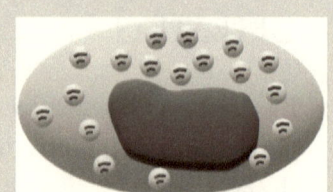

- Assembly of the viral components into a virus. This takes place either in the nucleus or cytoplasm.
- Non- enveloped viruses are present intracellularly as fully developed viruses.
- Enveloped viruses on the other hand have only the nucleocapsids ready. Their enveloped will later be derived from the host cell membrane as they are released.

RELEASE

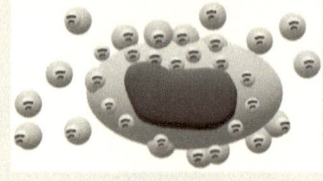

- The viruses are released from the cell by two means:

1. Either by rupturing the cell membrane thus killing the cell (mainly seen in non-enveloped viruses).
2. Or budding from the cell, using parts of the cell membrane as their envelope (seen in enveloped viruses).

- The newly made viruses are now free to infect more cells.

Since the host cell ended in death, this method of viral replication can be referred to as the *lytic cycle*. 'Lytic' is derived from the world 'lysis', which means the disintegration of a cell by rupture of its membrane or wall.

However, some viruses use an alternative pathway called the *lysogenic cycle.* In contrast to the lytic cycle, the lysogenic cycle does not end in the destruction of the host cell. In fact, the host cell acts as a sort of refuge for the virus as it lies dormant. The DNA of the virus integrates itself with the host cell chromosomes. The viral nucleic acid continues to function in its integrated state, conferring new properties to the host cell. No progeny is made at this point. Under stressful conditions, the viral DNA may be excised from the chromosome and the virus enters the lytic cycle.

Part 3: Classification of Viruses

The classification of viruses can be done based on two major criteria. Namely, its chemical and morphological properties. In other words, we can divide the viruses into several categories depending on the type of nucleic acid they contain or their capsid (size, symmetry and whether or not it is enveloped). For simplification, the following classification will be done under the heading of types of nucleic acid. Examples given under each subcategory are the names of virus families. Viruses which share similarities in morphology and nucleic acid fall under a family. Several examples of medically important viruses belonging to each family are listed below but will be further discussed in Part 4.

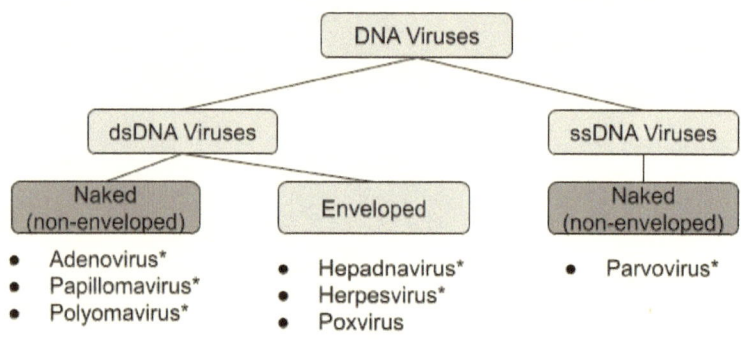

dsDNA : double stranded DNA
ssDNA : single stranded DNA
* icosahedral capsid

VIRUS FAMILY	EXAMPLES
Adenovirus	• Adenovirus
Papillomavirus	• Human papillomavirus (HPV)
Polyomavirus	• JC virus • BK virus

Hepadnavirus	• Hepatitis B virus (HBV)
Herpesvirus	• Herpes simplex virus (HSV) • Varicella zoster virus (VZV) • Cytomegalovirus (CMV) • Epstein-Barr Virus (EBV)
Poxvirus	• Smallpox • Molluscum contagiosum virus (MCV)
Parvovirus	• B19 virus

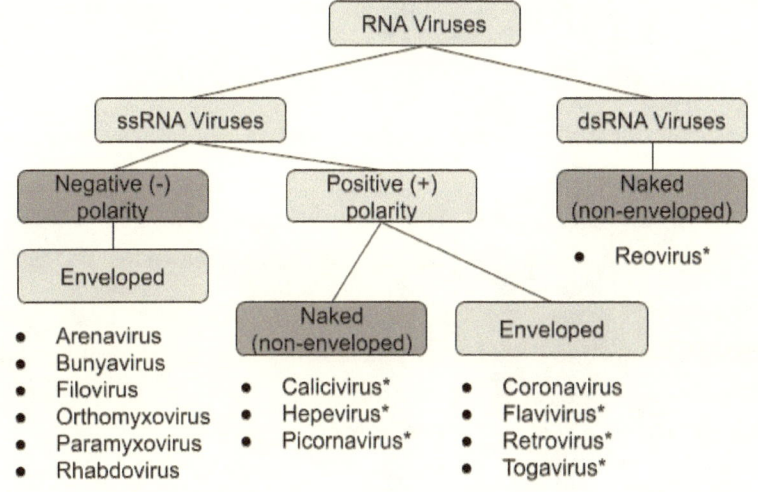

dsRNA : double stranded RNA
ssRNA : single stranded RNA
*icosahedral capsid

VIRUS FAMILY	EXAMPLES
Calicivirus	• Norovirus
Hepevirus	• Hepatitis E virus (HEV)
Picornavirus	• Poliovirus • Rhinovirus • Hepatitis A virus (HAV)
Coronavirus	• Covid-19
Flavivirus	• Yellow fever virus • Dengue virus • Hepatitis C virus (HCV) • West Nile virus
Retrovirus	• Human Immunodeficiency Virus (HIV) • Human T cell leukemia virus
Togavirus	• Rubella virus
Arenavirus	• Lassa fever • Lymphocytic choriomeningitis virus
Bunyavirus	• Hantavirus • California encephalitis virus
Filovirus	• Ebola virus • Marburg virus

Orthomyxovirus	• Influenza virus
Paramyxovirus	• Measles virus • Mumps virus • Respiratory syncytial virus • Nipah virus
Rhabdovirus	• Rabies virus
Reovirus	• Rotavirus
Deltavirus	• Hepatitis D virus (HDV)

Part 4: Medically Significant Viruses

There is no doubt that viruses have a greater potential to cause an epidemic or even a pandemic. This is due to the fact that the transmission of viruses across a population is more rapid compared to other pathogens. In 2015, the World Health Organization posted a list of top eight emerging diseases that are likely to cause an epidemic, all of which are of viral aetiologies (causative factor). However, this list is subjected to change based on the discovery of new diseases. Furthermore, certain viruses are capable of changing their antigenicity (further discussed under influenza virus below) so that any previous immunity developed against it may be rendered useless. This holds true especially for the flu viruses like the influenza virus.

Thus, it would be beneficial to get an idea of how certain clinically significant viruses transmit and the disease they cause.

DNA VIRUSES

1. HERPESVIRUSES:

VIRUS	TRANSMISSION	DISEASE	COMMENTS
Herpes Simplex Virus (HSV)	• HSV-1: Respiratory secretions and saliva • HSV-2: Sexual contact and perinatal infection (during delivery of foetus)	• HSV-1: Lesions above the waste - cold sores, keratitis, encephalitis • HSV-2: Lesions below the waist - genital herpes, neonatal encephalitis, neonatal herpes, meningitis	Divided into HSV type 1 (HSV-1) and HSV type 2 (HSV-2) Encephalitis is the inflammation of the brain tissue

Varicella Zoster Virus (VZV)	• Respiratory droplets • Direct contact with lesion	• Chickenpox • Shingles	
Cytomegalovirus (CMV)	• Cross placenta • Within the birth canal • Breast milk • Saliva • Sexual contact • Blood transfusion	• Congenital abnormalities in neonates • Pneumonia	
Epstein-Barr Virus (EBV)	Saliva	• Infectious mononucleosis • Lymphomas • Nasopharyngeal cancer	A.k.a. *Kissing disease* due to its mode of transmission

2. HEPADNAVIRUS:

VIRUS	TRANSMISSION	DISEASE	COMMENTS
Hepatitis B Virus (HBV)	• Blood products • Sexual intercourse • Perinatal infection (mother to newborn)	Viral Hepatitis	High risk behaviour: • Tattooing • Unprotected sex • Promiscuity • Needle sharing • Intravenous drug use

3. POXVIRUSES:

VIRUS	TRANSMISSION	DISEASE	COMMENTS
Smallpox Virus	• Respiratory aerosols • Direct contact with lesion or fomite	Smallpox	The only virus successfully eradicated from the world through vaccination programs
Molluscum Contagiosum Virus (MCV)	• Close contact • Sexual contact	Molluscum contagiosum	Common in children; manifest as painless, non-itchy, not inflamed flesh coloured papule on skin and mucous membrane

4. ADENOVIRUSES:

VIRUS	TRANSMISSION	DISEASE	COMMENTS
Adenovirus	• Respiratory droplets • Faecal-oral route • Finger-to-eye	• Pharyngitis (sore throat) • Conjunctivitis (pink eyes) • Common cold • Pneumonia	

5. PAPILLOMAVIRUS:

VIRUS	TRANSMISSION	DISEASE	COMMENTS
Human Papillomavirus (HPV)	• Skin to skin contact • Sexual contact	• Skin warts • Genital warts • Cervical cancer	More than a hundred types of papillomavirus.

6. PARVOVIRUS:

VIRUS	TRANSMISSION	DISEASE	COMMENTS
Parvovirus B19	• Respiratory route • Cross placenta • Blood transfusion	• Slapped cheek syndrome • Aplastic anaemia • Foetal infection	

RNA VIRUSES

1. ORTHOMYXOVIRUS:

VIRUS	TRANSMISSION	DISEASE	COMMENTS
Influenza virus	Airborne respiratory droplets	Influenza	

Influenza viruses can change their antigenicity and potentially cause devastating pandemics. They do so via two mechanisms: *antigenic shift* or *antigenic drift.*

Antigenic Shift:

- *Major change* based on *reassortment* of RNA
- Drastic and abrupt change in antigenic structure
- The new virus becomes unrelated to predecessor virus
- Antibodies developed against the predecessor virus fail to neutralize the new virus
- Potentially leads to a pandemic

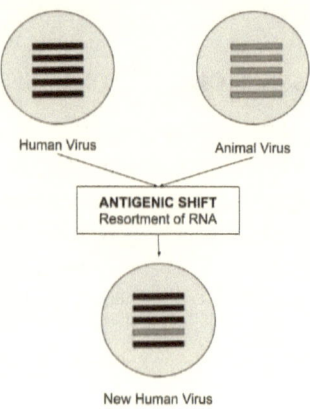

Antigenic drift:

- Minor change based on *mutation* of RNA
- Gradual and sequential change in antigenic structure
- Still related to predecessor virus
- Antibodies developed against predecessor virus effective against the new virus to varying extent
- Accounts for epidemics

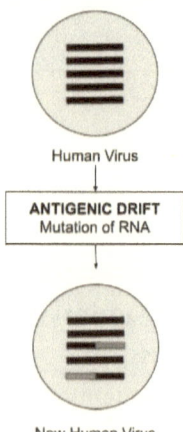

Pandemics and epidemics occur when the antigenicity of a virus changes to the extent that pre-existing immunity in many people are no longer effective against it.

2. PARAMYXOVIRUS:

VIRUS	TRANSMISSION	DISEASE	COMMENTS
Measles Virus	Respiratory droplets	Measles	
Mumps Virus	Respiratory droplets	• Mumps • Orchitis (inflammation of testes) • Meningitis	
Respiratory Syncytial Virus (RSV)	Respiratory droplets	• Bronchiolitis • Pneumonia	Common in children
Parainfluenza Virus	Respiratory droplet	• Croup • Bronchiolitis • Pneumonia	Common in children

3. CORONAVIRUS:

VIRUS	TRANSMISSION	DISEASE	COMMENTS
Coronaviruses	Respiratory aerosol	• Common cold • Severe acute respiratory syndrome (SARS) • Middle East respiratory syndrome (MERS)	The second most common flu viruses after the rhinovirus. The novel coronavirus named COVID-19 is responsible for the pandemic in 2020.

4. TOGAVIRUS:

VIRUS	TRANSMISSION	DISEASE	COMMENTS
Rubella Virus	• Respiratory droplet • Cross placenta	• Rubella • Congenital rubella syndrome	

5. RHABDOVIRUS:

VIRUS	TRANSMISSION	DISEASE	COMMENTS
Rabies Virus	Through bite of a rabid animal	Rabies (encephalitis)	

6. RETROVIRUS:

VIRUS	TRANSMISSION	DISEASE	COMMENTS
Human Immunodeficiency Virus (HIV)	• Sexual contact • Transfer of infected blood product • Perinatal transmission - cross placenta, at birth or breast milk	Acquired immunodeficiency syndrome (AIDS)	
Human T-cell Lymphocytic Virus (HTLV)	• Intravenous drug use • Sexual contact • Breast feeding	• Adult T-cell leukaemia • HTLV-associated myelopathy	Has 2 types: HTLV-1 and HTLV-2 which largely causes the same disease.

7. FILOVIRUS:

VIRUS	TRANSMISSION	DISEASE	COMMENTS
Ebola Virus	• Suspected natural reservoir of the virus: Fruit bats, monkeys • Human-to-human transmission: blood products and body fluid	Ebola haemorrhagic fever	
Marburg Virus	• Suspected natural reservoir of the virus: Bats	Haemorrhagic fever	

8. PICORNAVIRUS:

This family of viruses includes enteroviruses and rhinoviruses.

8.A Enteroviruses

VIRUS	TRANSMISSION	DISEASE	COMMENTS
Poliovirus	Faecal-oral route	Poliomyelitis	
Coxsackie Virus	• Faecal-oral route • Respiratory aerosol	• Herpangina • Acute haemorrhagic conjunctivitis • Hand-Foot-Mouth disease • Myocarditis (inflammation of the heart muscle) • Pericarditis • Pleurodynia (devil's grip) • Upper respiratory tract infection • Meningitis	

| Echovirus | Faecal-oral route | • Meningitis
 • Upper respiratory tract infection
 • Febrile illness
 • Infantile diarrhoea
 • Haemorrhagic conjunctivitis | |
| Hepatitis A Virus | Faecal-oral route | Viral Hepatitis | |

8.B Rhinovirus

VIRUS	TRANSMISSION	DISEASE	COMMENTS
Rhinovirus	• Respiratory droplets • Indirect via fomite	Common Cold	

9. CALICIVIRUS:

VIRUS	TRANSMISSION	DISEASE	COMMENTS
Norovirus	• Faecal-oral route • Ingestion of contaminated seafood or water	Gastroenteritis	

10. REOVIRUS:

VIRUS	TRANSMISSION	DISEASE	COMMENTS
Rotavirus	Faecal-oral route	Viral gastroenteritis	Common in children

HEPATITIS VIRUSES

VIRUS	FAMILY	TRANSMISSION	DISEASE	COMMENTS
Hepatitis A Virus	Picornavirus	Faecal-oral route	Viral hepatitis	Vaccine available
Hepatitis B Virus	Hepadnavirus	• Blood • Sex • At birth	Viral hepatitis	Vaccine available
Hepatitis C Virus	Flavivirus	• Blood • Sex	Viral hepatitis	
Hepatitis D Virus	Deltavirus	• Blood • Sex	Viral hepatitis	
Hepatitis E Virus	Hepevirus	Faecal-oral route	Viral hepatitis	

ARBOVIRUS

Viruses spread via insects. The word *arbo* is short for *arthropod-borne*.

VIRUS	FAMILY	TRANSMISSION	DISEASE
Dengue Virus	Flavivirus	Via mosquito	• Classic dengue fever • Dengue haemorrhagic fever
Yellow Fever Virus	Flavivirus	Via mosquito	Yellow fever
West Nile Virus	Flavivirus	Via mosquito	• Encephalitis • meningitis

Japanese Encephalitis Virus (JE virus)	Flavivirus	Via mosquito	Encephalitis
Chikungunya Virus	Togavirus	Via mosquito	• Arthralgia (joint pain) • Rash • Encephalitis
Nipah Virus	Paramyxovirus	• Natural reservoir: fruit bats, pigs • Human-to-human transmission via saliva, sputum (phlegm)	Encephalitis

Part 5: How Antiviral Drugs Work?

In contrast to the wide array of medications that can be prescribed to patients suffering an infection of bacterial origin, there are not many antiviral drugs out in the market. This is because there is difficulty in finding an agent with a selective (specific) toxicity towards viruses as their replication process is largely integrated with the normal processes of its host cell.

However, there are a few classes of antiviral drugs that are approved for use. The principle of antiviral therapy, like antibiotics or antifungal drugs, are aimed at disrupting the normal processes so that there is failure of replication and/or spread.

MECHANISM OF ACTION OF ANTIVIRAL DRUGS WITH EXAMPLES:

1. Inhibition of early events which includes entry and uncoating of the virus.

   Example: Amantadine

   Rimantadine

   Maraviroc

2. Inhibition of nucleic acid synthesis.

   <u>For Herpesviruses</u>

   Example: Acyclovir

   Ganciclovir

   <u>For Human Immunodeficiency Virus (HIV)</u>

   A combination of drugs are needed to control HIV. This is popularly known as Highly Active Antiretroviral Therapy or HAART for short.

   Example: Zidovudine

   Lamivudine

   Emtricitabine

   Abacavir

> Tenofovir
> Nevirapine

For Hepatitis B Virus (HBV)
Example: Adefovir

     Lamivudine

     Tenofovir

Others:
Example: Ribavirin

3. Inhibits the release of influenza virus from an infected cell
  Example: Oseltamivir

      Zanamivir

4. Inhibition of protein synthesis
  Example: Interferon

      Fomivirsen

Despite the availability of such antiviral drugs, its use is very limited. Viral replication mostly occurs during the incubation period where the patient is still well. By the time symptoms manifest and a diagnosis is made, it may be ineffective to administer these drugs as the virus has already spread throughout the body. That's why doctors don't normally give antiviral medication when patients have chickenpox, measles or mumps for instance, and allow the disease to just run its course. We are fortunate to have an immune system strong enough to overcome these diseases. Then again, getting vaccinated in the first place helps our immune system better prepare itself and widely reduces mortality. There are certain exceptions where antiviral therapy must be initiated as soon as a diagnosis is made (e.g. hepatitis, HIV) and may be required to continue lifelong to stop or retard the progress of the disease (e.g. HIV).

Another challenge for antiviral therapy is the emergence of drug-resistant viruses. Hence, a combination of drugs of different mechanisms of action must be used to avoid therapeutic failure.

Prevention is always better than cure. We have come to learn the various ways viruses can transmit. By taking simple measures, we can prevent ourselves from contracting them in the first place, sparing us the trouble of having to endure through the symptoms of the disease and consuming multiple medications. Viruses that spread via respiratory droplets can be stopped by wearing a mask when sick. Those that transmit through faecal-oral routes can be easily avoided by properly washing and cooking food coupled with handwashing before meals. Arthropod-borne viruses can be mitigated by using mosquito repellents, mosquito netting, and destroying breeding hotspots.

Basic Virology Summary

- Viruses are neither alive nor dead. However, they require a living cell as a host to replicate, utilizing its biological machinery to make copies of itself.
- Viral replication often results in the death of its host cell (lytic cycle). Sometimes, they infect a cell and remain dormant in it (lysogenic cycle) until a point in the future where they reactivate and enter the lytic cycle.
- Viruses can be classified in various ways, but the two main classifications are based on the type of nucleic acid they harbour or based on their morphology (structure).
- Viruses that can cause human diseases are of medical importance and a good number of them have been listed in Part 4.
- Antiviral medications are not often used in practice. There are exceptions to the rule (e.g. HIV, hepatitis etc).

FOOD FOR THOUGHT:

Viruses and bacteria aren't the best of friends. They have been engaged in war for millions of years. Viruses that attack bacteria are known as bacteriophages. By studying their battles, scientists were able to pick up a few things that could benefit mankind. For example, bacteria developed a defence mechanism against viruses that allowed them to identify and 'snip off' viral nucleic acid from their chromosome using the CRISPR/Cas system. The expanded form of CRISPR is *clustered regularly interspaced short palindromic repeats*. It can be used as a gene editing tool. Imagine using CRISPR to snip off defective genes and using a virus as a vehicle to integrate desired genes into a cell. Genetic diseases could be a thing of the past. This opens up a multitude of gateways in the field of genetic engineering. Furthermore, bacteriophages can be used where antibiotics fail. This is known as *phage therapy*. Here, viruses are used against antibiotic-resistant infections to help cure patients. There have already been several instances where phage therapy was used successfully. However, more research in this direction is still required though the road ahead is promising. In the trying times of a pandemic, viruses seem to only give off a sense of devastation and despair. Situations can turn from bad to worse so fast it seems like God may have created it for the sole purpose of punishment. When you see it that way, it does sound like monsters from horror stories. It *is* neither dead nor alive. But we must learn not to be quick in judgment. Viruses, in all their uniqueness, bring with them new fields of research and applications that the human race can use to its advantage.

CHAPTER 9

Basic Parasitology

The study of parasites

Part 1: Characteristics and Classification of Parasites
Part 2: Medically Significant Parasites and Antiparasitic Drugs

·

Summary

Part 1: Characteristics and Classification of Parasites

When we think of parasites, the thought of one thing feeding off another usually comes to mind. Sometimes, people use it as an insult to describe others that are taking advantage of somebody else. By definition, a parasite is an organism that is entirely dependent on another organism, living on it or in it, for all stages of its life cycle and metabolic requirements.

There are two classes of parasites that can cause disease in humans. They are *protozoa* and *helminths* (otherwise called worms). The Centers for Disease Control and Prevention (CDC) categorize them under three headings. Namely, protozoa, helminths and ectoparasite. If you recall, protozoa fall under the kingdom Protista.

Picture the following scenario, it is almost New Year's Day and you decide to clean and spruce up the house a little. You've neglected the mess you've made for quite a while and decided it's high time you keep things organized. So, you got a few boxes and labelled them according to the stuff that falls under the same category. For instance, magazines go into one box, trash goes into another and your kid's toys back into the toy basket. At the end of the day, you find that there are several items that don't fit into any category that you came up with. You then decided to open up a new box, labelled it 'miscellaneous' and dumped them all in. That's basically what the kingdom Protista is. A bunch of misfits that don't seem to fit into the other four kingdoms of life. Protists are eukaryotic organisms that cannot be classified as either bacteria, fungi, animals or plants. Protists refer to the members of the kingdom Protista. They include protozoa.

Protista is the Greek word for 'the very first'. It was named as such because protists were thought to be the first eukaryotic form of life, predecessor to multicellular eukaryotes in the kingdoms Plantae, Animalia and Fungi. Most protist species are unicellular organisms with exceptions such as kelp. Kelps are multicellular protists. Some species of kelp can even grow over a hundred feet in height.

However, the topic of interest that we shall be discussing under this kingdom is the microparasite, protozoa. All protozoa share the following properties:

- They are all a unicellular organism
- They are a eukaryotic cell. This means they have membrane bounded organelles such as mitochondria, Golgi apparatus, endoplasmic reticulum, a nucleus with nuclear membrane etc.
- They can perform all functions of life such as respiration, digestion, excretion, reproduction and locomotion.
- They possess organs of locomotion. Based on this feature, they can be subclassified into *amoebas, sporozoans, flagellates* and *ciliates*. (Refer diagram below)
- They reproduce asexually.

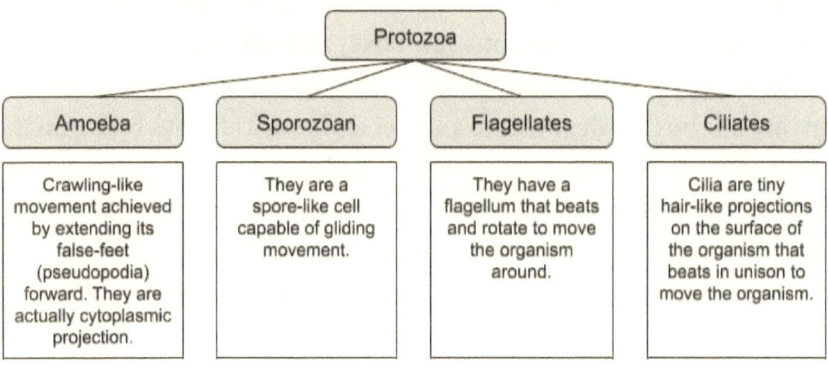

On the other hand, helminths a.k.a. worms are large, multicellular organisms that are generally visible to the naked eye when in adult form. Adult helminths cannot reproduce inside the human body. Similar to protozoa, they are further subdivided into three classes: *cestodes, nematodes* and *trematodes*.

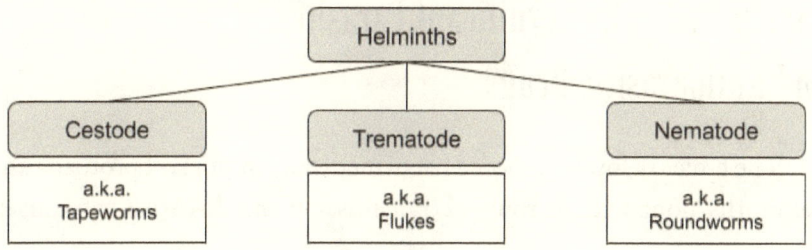

The CDC refers to ectoparasites as organisms like ticks, fleas, lice, and mites that attach or burrow into the skin and remain there for relatively long periods of time (e.g. weeks to months). However, it could broadly include arthropods like mosquitos. But they bear more significance as vectors/transmitters of diseases.

Part 2: Medically Significant Parasites and Antiparasitic Drugs

The tables below will show a list of medically important protozoa and helminths along with its route of transmission and disease it can cause.

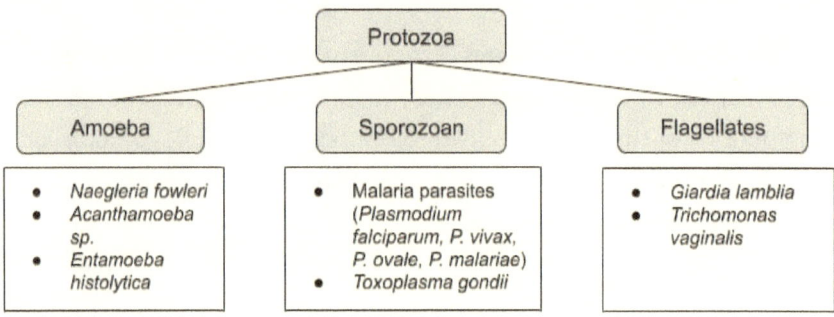

PROTOZOA:

PROTOZOAL SPECIES	TRANSMISSION	DISEASE
Naegleria fowleri a.k.a the 'brain eating' parasite.	• They are ubiquitous in soil and water • Swimming in chlorinated pools, lakes and ponds	Primary amoebic meningoencephalitis (PAM) • Inflammation of the meninges and brain tissue.
Acanthamoeba sp.	• Inhalation of aerosol and dust • Invasion through broken/ulcerated skin or eyes	Granulomatous amoebic encephalitis (GAE)

Entamoeba histolytica	• Ingested through faecal-oral route	Amoebic dysentery (bloody diarrhoea)
Malaria parasites	• Mosquito bite	Malaria
Toxoplasma gondii	• Ingestion of contaminated water or undercooked meat	Toxoplasma encephalitis
Giardia lamblia	• Faecal-oral route	Diarrhoea Steatorrhea (presence of fat in stool making it oily white and foul-smelling)
Trichomonas vaginalis	• Sexual intercourse	Vaginitis (inflammation of vagina)

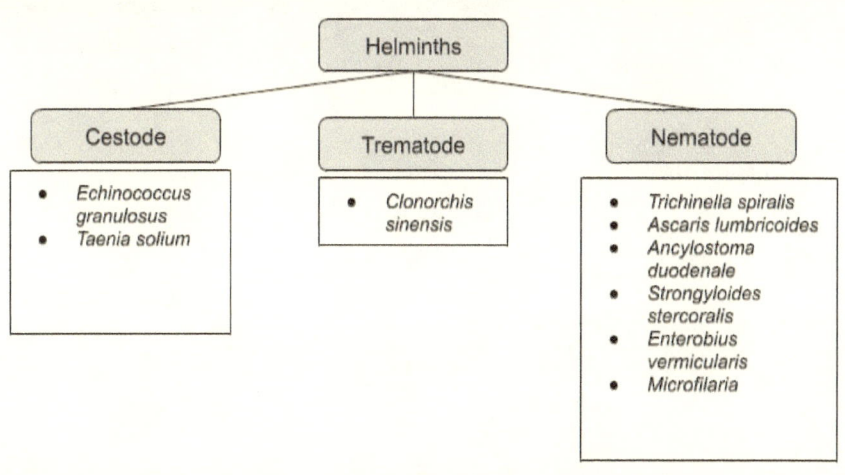

HELMINTHS:

HELMINTH SPECIES	TRANSMISSION	DISEASE
Echinococcus granulosus a.k.a dog tapeworm/ hydatid worm	• Direct contact with infected dogs • Allowing dogs to feed from same dish as humans • Ingestion of contaminated food and water	• Liver: chronic abdominal pain • Lung: cough, shortness of breath, chest pain • Allergic reaction
Taenia solium a.k.a. pork tapeworm	• Ingestion of undercooked pork containing larvae • Ingestion of contaminated water and food	• Diarrhoea • Headache • Vomiting • Brain involvement: seizure, behavioural changes • Eye involvement: inflammation
Clonorchis sinensis a.k.a. liver flukes	• Ingestion of raw, undercooked, salted or pickled freshwater fish	• Abdominal distress • Diarrhoea • Bile duct cancer

Trichinella spiralis	• Ingestion of undercooked meat	• Diarrhoea • Vomiting • Abdominal pain • Muscle pain • Fatigue
Ascaris lumbricoides	• Faecal-oral route	• Malnutrition • Abdominal pain • Intestinal pain or perforation • Pancreatitis • Allergic reaction • Worms coming out of unusual orifices e.g. ear, anus, nose etc.
Ancylostoma duodenale a.k.a. hookworm	• Penetration of skin • Usually walking barefoot on soil	• Ground itch (on foot) • Iron deficiency anaemia
Strongyloides stercoralis	• Penetration of skin • Usually walking barefoot on soil	• Dermatitis • Itching • Pneumonia • Bloating • Diarrhoea • Malabsorption syndrome • Stomach ulcer • Dysentery (bloody diarrhoea)

Enterobius vermicularis	• Faecal-oral route • Self-infection: anus- hands- mouth • Inhalation of eggs in disturbed clothes, bedding, dust	• Itching in area of anus • Vaginitis • Appendicitis • Urine incontinence • Weight loss
Microfilaria (*Wuchereria bancrofti*)	• Mosquito bite	• Elephantiasis

Most of the parasitic infection transmitted by ingestion can be easily avoided by ensuring food hygiene and making sure everything is cooked properly.

There are drugs that can be prescribed to treat patients suffering from parasitic infection. Their mechanism of actions are described as follows:

1. Antiamoebic drugs:
    Damages microbial DNA leading to death of organism
    Example: Metronidazole
          Secnidazole
          Tinidazole

2. Anthelmintic drugs
    A) Breakdown of cytoplasmic microtubules (component of cytoskeleton), inhibits glucose uptake by organism, depletes glycogen storage and disrupts metabolic pathways of parasites.
    Example: Mebendazole
          Albendazole

B) Results in the intense contraction of the musculature of the parasite, causing it to become paralysed and eventually passed out in stool.

Creates holes in the parasite for the immune system to kill it more effectively.

Example: Praziquantel

C) Cause blood vessel vasoconstriction to impair passage of microfilariae.

Alters the membrane of microfilariae for the immune system to work against it more effectively.

Example: Diethylcarbamazine citrate (DEC)

3. Antimalarial drugs

Disrupts metabolic pathway of the malarial parasite.

Example: Chloroquine
                Mefloquine
                Primaquine
                Doxycycline
                Artesunate
                Artemether

Basic Parasitology Summary

- Parasites are organisms that fully depend on its host to survive.
- Parasites can be unicellular (protozoa) or multicellular (helminths).
- Protozoa are eukaryotic cells which are further subclassified by their locomotion into amoebas, sporozoans, flagellates and ciliates.
- Helminths are subclassified into nematodes, trematodes and cestodes.
- Parasites that can cause human diseases are of medical importance and a good number of them have been listed in Part 2.
- There are a few categories of antiparasitic drugs that are available to treat patients suffering from an infection.

FOOD FOR THOUGHT:

Parasites, by definition, are bad for the host. If there's anything that we can learn from them, it would be 'Adapt to Survive'. From the beginning of life on earth, not all organisms turned out to be able to fend for themselves and survive. This is where parasites have evolved to feed off a host, letting it do all the hard work. This may not be a very good value to impart but the awareness of how nature finds a way, even for its weakest offspring, is simply fascinating and worth beholding.

CHAPTER 10

"If you do not study life, it makes no sense" - Plato

O ur planet is a peculiar place in the cosmos. Through the incomprehensible vastness of interstellar space, we find a lonely pile of dirt floating around the galactic habitable zone of the Milky Way harbouring organisms. This tiny spec of a planet in some forgotten corner of the universe holds what probably is the only gem of creation, intelligent life.

But it was not always like that. We humans, now at the brink of knowledge, came from humble beginnings. Our origins were nothing larger than a single cell. Isn't it just fascinating to contemplate that the evolution of life came so far that it is almost impossible to fathom that such complexities of the human body stemmed from just a simple prokaryote. This notion begs for another question, how can something non-living when put together in certain combination make something alive? Maybe even conscious? I find this to be a beautiful mystery. If there wasn't a divine creator out there, then our existence must be a grand accident of one event leading to another. Whatever your beliefs may be, isn't it wonderful to be part of evolution and development, the greatest show on earth. Hence, we must be grateful for how far we have journeyed together in time, bringing along all forms of life into the world.

It is with this epiphany that my love for science began to grow ever since I was a young boy. My fascination for life landed me in the state library almost every weekend during my childhood, reading and learning about space, time and evolution. Throughout my studies, I have understood one thing. It is the smallest things which define the big picture. Hence, my choice in presenting you a book about microscopic life. I came to realize that certain concepts of life can be derived from this subject in helping us re-evaluate ourselves and rethink our place in the cosmos. My objective is to make you aware and appreciate the uniqueness of our existence and the extraordinary journey life has undertaken to bring you to this time and place so that we won't take our daily living for granted. Learning about life beginning from the womb is merely touching the surface of the matter. That is the reason I did my level best to incorporate some personal thoughts into the chapters of this book. To me, simply knowing is not enough, we must also appreciate. Knowledge can make us arrogant, but appreciation humbles a person.

With this understanding, we now know with certainty that all life is related. From the tiniest insect to the largest whale, we are all offsprings of the same tree of life. The same matter used in the first mammal is the exact building blocks that make us human. There's this invisible thread that binds us all together as one tree of life. Doesn't it sadden you looking at how some humans in their petty struggle for wealth and power treat their own kind in the way that they do? To satisfy the greed of man, nature too has been exploited in hideous ways. We must not be ignorant to the fact that our actions impact the delicate bond between life on earth. I sincerely hope that after going through this book, you may have a different outlook and perspective of life and be mindful of your actions. It's a small world after all.

As inhabitants of earth, we are moving forward. This means that we have passed certain sign posts and will continue to pass more sign posts in the future. The first was creation of life, then intelligent life. We even left Earth for the moon. What next? Just like many visionaries, I too believe that our future lies in the stars. Someday, perhaps a few hundred years from now, our descendants will look back on this home planet and reflect upon their humble genesis, from a world once only observable under the microscope.

Jesper Leonard Vun

BIBLIOGRAPHY

Ahmadjian, V, Alexopoulos, CJ & Moore, D 2020, *Fungus,* Viewed 24 April 2020, https://www.britannica.com/science/fungus

Basic Biology 2018, *Tree of Life,* Viewed 17 April 2020, https://basicbiology.net/biology-101/tree-of-life

Basic Biology 2019, *Taxonomy,* Viewed 12 April 2020, https://basicbiology.net/biology-101/taxonomy

Berger, K 2019, *Alexander Fleming and the Discovery of Penicillin,* Viewed 16 April 2020, https://www.pharmacytimes.com/contributor/karen-berger/2019/03/alexander-fleming-and-the-discovery-of-penicillin

BYJU's The Learning App n.d., *Kingdom Fungi,* Viewed 24 April 2020, https://byjus.com/biology/kingdom-fungi/

BYJU's The Learning App n.d., *Protista,* Viewed 26 July 2020, https://byjus.com/biology/protista/

Carr, S 2011, *Five Kingdoms vs. Three Domains,* Viewed 15 April 2020, https://www.mun.ca/biology/scarr/Five_Kingdoms_Three_Domains.html

Charles Darwin and the Tree of Life. (2009). [Online]. Produced by Brian Leith. United Kingdom: BBC One [Viewed 27 March 2020]. Available from Amazon Prime.

Centers for Disease Control and Prevention 2020, *Serotypes and the Importance of Serotyping Salmonella,* Viewed 16 April 2020, https://www.cdc.gov/salmonella/reportspubs/salmonella-atlas/serotyping-importance.html

Centers for Disease Control and Prevention 2016, *About Parasites,* Viewed 26 July 2020, https://www.cdc.gov/parasites/about.html#ecto

Centers for Disease Control and Prevention 2021, *Understanding How the COVID-19 Vaccine Work,* Viewed 21 January 2021, https://www.cdc.gov/coronavirus/2019-ncov/vaccines/different-vaccines/how-they-work.html

Daley, J 2017, *How Microscopic Algae Kick-Started Life As We Know It,* Viewed 24 April 2020, https://www.smithsonianmag.com/smart-news/how-oceans-algae-and-huge-snowball-led-complex-life-180964567/

Fox, A 2019, *Viruses Genetically Engineered to Kill Bacteria Rescues Girl With Antibiotic-resistant Infection,* Viewed 25 July 2020, https://www.sciencemag.org/news/2019/05/viruses-genetically-engineered-kill-bacteria-rescue-girl-antibiotic-resistant-infection

Gan, WY 2013, *Success Biology SPM,* Oxford Fajar Sdn. Bhd., Shah Alam, Selangor Darul Ehsan.

Greene, A 2010, *Bacteria vs. Viruses,* Viewed 25 July 2020, https://www.drgreene.com/qa-articles/bacteria-vs-viruses

Hanley, K 2011, *The double-edged sword: How evolution can make or break a live-attenuated virus vaccine. Evolution*, 4(4), 635–643. https://doi.org/10.1007/s12052-011-0365-y

Healthline 2016, *The Most Dangerous Epidemics in U.S. History*, Viewed 16 April 2020, https://www.healthline.com/health/worst-disease-outbreaks-history#1

History.com editors, 2010, *Jenner Tests Smallpox Vaccines*, Viewed 5 April 2020, https://www.history.com/this-day-in-history/jenner-tests-smallpox-vaccine

Iftikhar, N 2019, *What is Phage Therapy?*, Viewed 25 July 2020, https://www.healthline.com/health/phage-therapy

Lakna 2017, *Difference Between Algae and Fungi*, Viewed 24 April 2020, https://pediaa.com/difference-between-algae-and-fungi/

Le, T, Bhushan, V, Sochat, M & Vaidyanathan, V 2020, *First Aid For The USMLE Step 1 International Edition*, McGraw Hill Education, USA.

Levin, R.A. & Anderson, R.A. 2019, *Algae*, Viewed 24 April 2020, https://www.britannica.com/science/algae/Physical-and-ecological-features-of-algae

Levinson, W 2016, *Review of Medical Microbiology and Immunology, Fourteenth Edition*, McGraw-Hill Education, United States of America.

LibreTexts 2019, *Types of Microorganism*, Viewed 20 April 2020, https://bio.libretexts.org/Bookshelves/Microbiology/Book%3A_Microbiology_(Boundless)/1%3A_Introduction_to_Microbiology/1.2%3A_Microbes_and_the_World/1.2A_Types_of_Microorganisms

Lumen Boundless Microbiology n.d., *Viral Replication*, Viewed 22 July 2020, https://courses.lumenlearning.com/boundless-microbiology/chapter/viral-replication/

Lumen Learning Microbiology n.d., *Characteristics of Infectious Disease,* Viewed 16 April 2020, https://courses.lumenlearning.com/microbiology/chapter/characteristics-of-infectious-disease/

Lumen Learning Microbiology n.d., *Classification of Fungi,* Viewed 24 April 2020, *https://courses.lumenlearning.com/biology2xmaster/chapter/classification-of-fungi/*

Lumen Learning Microbiology n.d., *Fungi,* Viewed 24 April 2020, https://courses.lumenlearning.com/microbiology/chapter/fungi/

Lumen Learning Microbiology n.d., *Importance of Fungi in Human Life,* Viewed 28 April 2020, https://courses.lumenlearning.com/boundless-biology/chapter/importance-of-fungi-in-human-life/

Microscope Master 2019, *Difference Between Serotype, Strain and Genotype,* Viewed 16 April 2020, https://www.microscopemaster.com/serotype.html

Ochmann, S & Roser, M 2020, *Smallpox,* Viewed 5 April 2020, https://ourworldindata.org/smallpox

Rachna, C 2017, *Difference Between Prokaryotic Cells and Eukaryotic Cells,* Viewed 15 April 2020, https://biodifferences.com/difference-between-prokaryotic-cells-and-eukaryotic-cells.html

Rachna, C 2018, *Difference Between Archaea and Bacteria,* Viewed 15 April 2020, https://biodifferences.com/difference-between-archaea-and-bacteria.html#Conclusion

Sharma, H, Sharma, K 2017, *Principles of Pharmacology,* Paras Medical Publisher, Hyderabad

Sen, A 2018, *How a Battle Between Bacteria and Viruses is Being Used For Human Health,* Viewed 25 July 2020, https://science.thewire.in/the-sciences/how-a-battleground-between-bacteria-and-viruses-is-being-used-for-human-health/

Steward, K 2018, *Lytic vs Lysogenic - Understanding Bacteriophage Life Cycles*, Viewed 22 July 2020, https://www.technologynetworks.com/immunology/articles/lytic-vs-lysogenic-understanding-bacteriophage-life-cycles-308094

Study.com n.d., *Kingdom Protista: Definition, Characteristics & Examples*, Viewed 26 July 2020, https://study.com/academy/lesson/kingdom-protista-definition-characteristics-examples.html

UCMP Berkeley n.d., *Carl Linnaeus*, Viewed 12 April 2020, https://ucmp.berkeley.edu/history/linnaeus.html

Vaccine.gov 2020, *Vaccine Types*, Viewed 5 April 2020, https://www.vaccines.gov/basics/types

Villarreal, L 2008, *Are Viruses Alive? - Scientific American*, Viewed 21 July 2020, https://www.scientificamerican.com/article/are-viruses-alive-2004/

World Health Organization 2015, *WHO Publishes List of Top Emerging Diseases Likely To Cause Major Epidemics*, Viewed 25 July 2020, https://www.who.int/medicines/ebola-treatment/WHO-list-of-top-emerging-diseases/en/

Yeong, M L 2015, *Immunization schedule*, Viewed 20 January 2020, http://www.myhealth.gov.my/en/immunisation-schedule/

www.ingramcontent.com/pod-product-compliance
Lightning Source LLC
Chambersburg PA
CBHW020514290526
45786CB00002B/598